Praise for *Cereal for Dinner*

"*Cereal for Dinner* is a wonderful book packed with information for moms who are ill. It's upbeat, informative, and filled with Kristine's wisdom and insight. This is a must read for moms battling illness. I couldn't put it down."
—Elise Babcock, author of *When Life Becomes Precious: The Essential Guide for Patients, Loved Ones, and Friends of Those Facing Serious Illnesses*

"Mothers so often neglect themselves as they care for all those around them. This book will fill a critical gap, as it will teach women how to ask for help, accept help, and focus on their healing. Kristine's experience, suffering and recovering from a serious heart condition while caring for her two young kids, gives her a great platform from which to share these lessons."
—Noel Bairey Merz, M.D., Medical Director, Women's Health, Cedars-Sinai Medical Center, Los Angeles

"Kristine Breese's book is a much-needed guide for all women—and especially for mothers struggling through a difficult time in their own lives, due to health or other challenges. Who else is going to put us first if we don't do it for ourselves?"
—Michelle Morris-Spieker, author of *The Cherished Self*

"*Cereal for Dinner* is a book for everyone to read, including physicians."
—Ismael Nuno, M.D., Chief of Cardiothoracic Surgery, L.A. County and USC Medical Centers and Member of the Board, American Heart Association, Western States Affiliate

"*Cereal for Dinner* gently and lovingly gives baby-step by baby-step directions to families who have temporarily lost their way, when Mom suddenly becomes too ill to lead them forward. It is the perfect 'get well' gift for mothers battling illness, and by reading it they will soon have Kristine Breese, who channels the delightful humor and hard-won wisdom of Erma Bombeck, as their new best friend."
—Jacquelin Gorman, author of *The Seeing Glass* and former UCLA Medical Center Chaplain Intern

CEREAL
for DINNER

CEREAL *for* DINNER

STRATEGIES, SHORTCUTS, AND SANITY FOR MOMS BATTLING ILLNESS

Kristine Breese

 St. Martin's Griffin ❧ New York

www.stmartins.com

Excerpt from *The Hope Tree* reprinted with the permission of Simon & Schuster Books for Young Readers, an imprint of Simon & Schuster Children's Publishing Division. Copyright © 1999 Laura Numeroff and Wendy S. Harpham, M.D.

Excerpt from *Can I Still Kiss You?* reprinted with the permission of Health Communications, Inc. Copyright © 2001 Neil Russell.

Excerpt from *It Won't Hurt Forever: Guiding Your Child Through Trauma* used with permission from Peter Levine, Ph.D., from an audio program produced by Sounds True © 2001. www.soundstrue.com.

Excerpt from *Reflections in the Light* reprinted with the permission of New World Library, Novato, CA. www.newworldlibrary.com. Copyright © 1988 Shakti Gawain.

ISBN 0-312-31773-5
EAN 978-0312-31773-7

First Edition: May 2004

10 9 8 7 6 5 4 3 2 1

For Justus, Addison, and Travis

In Memory of
Louise Frova Swancoat and Mary Ellen Hagerman

CONTENTS

ACKNOWLEDGMENTS

The people who helped create this book fall into five categories.

The first group includes those who gave me life. In this group are, first and foremost, my parents, who have always believed in me and who cared for me even when I didn't know how to care for myself. Those who gave me life a second time, through use of shrewd minds and caring hands, are Dr. John Armato, Dr. Bruce Jackson, and Dr. Bruce Goldreyer. And then there's Jenny, who fits in here because she made the call that changed everything.

Those who enrich my life are the second group, and they include Judy, Teri, Joanna, May, and Lynne, who watched the kids so I could write—and cheered me on as I did. My life has also been enriched by three author/moms, Jennie, Jackie, and Michelle, who shared freely of what they know about both these demanding careers and whose input made the words ring true.

Those who share my life, Justus, Addison, and Travis, are the third group—and they are the reason this story matters.

Next are the eighteen moms who shared their stories so others might be helped, and to whom I am deeply indebted. This book is but a vessel and I am honored to carry it.

Finally, thanks go to my agent, Julie Castiglia, who took my call and listened to my two-minute pitch when I have since learned that agents *never* do that; to my editor, Heather Jackson, who got what this book was about and believed in it from the beginning, and her assistant, Elizabeth Bewley, who stepped in and made a difference with sparkling syntax and spirit.

FOREWORD

When I was a child, there was something wonderful about being sick. My mother was not normally the type of mom who would hover, coddle, and indulge, but when I was sick, she would bring home new coloring books, let me watch as many cartoons as I wanted, and blend magical, healing smoothies of pineapple juice and lime sherbet. Sure, I may have had a fever, a rash, or a stomach in revolt, but I also had my mom, without doubt and without interruption.

When I became a mother myself, and took on the responsibility for coddling, indulging, and protecting my children from all physical, spiritual, and emotional harm, the pleasure of my being sick evaporated like summer rain on a hot sidewalk. There was no longer anything good about having a sore throat or the flu, because now *I* was the one who was supposed to be doing the caretaking, and sickness just got in the way; it wasn't part of the natural order of things.

The idea of a sickness even worse than the flu—something debilitating, dangerous, perhaps even deadly—had no place whatsoever in my plans or my imagination, until, out of the blue, I was diagnosed with breast cancer at the age of thirty-five, when my kids were three and six, and I faced a long season of surgeries and complications. Among the many other difficult things I had to do was to reconstruct my notion of what it meant to be a mom. It didn't mean cook, clean, repair, find, fix, and bring coloring books home when the kids had a fever. It meant just being there and loving my kids more than anyone else was able.

As beautiful as this might sound in theory, it was really difficult to live out every day. I kept wishing for a guidebook on how to let go of what I couldn't do for my kids, while still holding on to what I alone could be to them.

That's where this book comes in. In *Cereal for Dinner*, Kristine Breese shows moms who are facing serious illnesses of all kinds just what to expect, and just how to deal with it, in practical, real-life, everyday ways. She talks about the nitty-gritty stuff like how much to tell the kids, how to know who to ask for help, what to do about the nagging guilt, how to think about the possibility of death, and the fact that, yeah, sometimes it's going to be cereal for dinner. She helps moms who are sick reconstruct their own notions of motherhood to accommodate the illness none of them ever planned for or imagined.

This book is, in other words, an enormous gift for any mom who finds herself sick. A big part of that gift is Kristine herself. I have the great pleasure of being her friend and colleague, and I can tell you that she is one of the wisest, most compassionate, upbeat, go-getter, inspiring people you'd ever want to know, and she has put a huge part of herself right here on the page. She is like your best mom-friend, who just happens to have a pacemaker; who just happens to have the experience of riding in ambulances while the kids stand on the curb waving good-bye; of waiting for test results while figuring out what everyone's going to be for Halloween; and of going flat-line in the exam room and having to face exactly what it means to be someone's mom *right here* and *right now*, in whatever condition you happen to find yourself. Kristine is leaning in close, in this book, telling it like it really is, and passing on a hope so bright it lights up the whole sky.

You'd be blessed, I believe, to listen.

—Jennie Nash, author of *The Victoria's Secret Catalog Never Stops Coming and Other Lessons I Learned from Breast Cancer*, and of *Raising a Reader: A Mother's Tale of Desperation and Delight*.

But you don't have to do anything, Mommy.
Just let me stay near you and we can talk,
and we can just be together like always.

—Jacquelin Gorman, *The Seeing Glass*

INTRODUCTION

What Happened to Me and How It Can Help You

I'd just come to after collapsing on the floor of the bathroom and all I could think of was macaroni and cheese. Jenny, my sister-in-law, was kneeling over me and telling me that the paramedics were on their way, but I would have none of that.

"I can't go to the hospital, the kids haven't had dinner yet," I offered up, thinking that would take care of everything. "I think there's some macaroni and cheese in the freezer."

I didn't want to be sick and didn't think I was. I had things to do and people counting on me, from hungry kids to unhappy clients. I wanted desperately for everything to be okay and life to go on as it had before.

But that day was the beginning of the end of mommy-life as I knew it.

◦   ◦   ◦

Starting in 1989 and continuing until my collapse in 1999, I had a series of fainting spells that I completely ignored. In fact, I

passed out ten times in the ten years before I ever saw a doctor—
and when I finally did go it was under protest and in an ambulance on the night Jenny called 911. Prior to that, I never sought
help and I always had excuses. I fainted on the subway in
Chicago and I attributed it to the muggy summer weather. It
happened waiting in the valet line in front of a Beverly Hills
restaurant and I assumed it was caused by something I'd eaten. It
happened on my wedding night and I wrote it off as nerves and
exhaustion. I did such a good job convincing everyone that I was
fine that even my mom had stopped asking me if I was going to
go to the doctor and find out why I "kept passing out."

But this all changed the night of September 15, 1999.

I had just arrived home after working late, and as my husband, Justus, was out of town Jenny was baby-sitting, having
taken over for the nanny who left at six o'clock. On the way
home, I started to feel queasy. As I drove I loosened the zipper on
my suit skirt. At the next stoplight I wriggled out of my panty
hose. Not too much farther, I reminded myself, and so I just focused on driving safely and getting there as quickly as possible.
When I arrived, I rushed past Jenny and the kids with a quick
hello and made a beeline for the bathroom. I told Jenny I was
feeling funny and asked her to stay a minute until it had passed.
The kids were engrossed in a *Jungle Book* video and Mogli was
still roaming around the forest with his bear and jaguar pals, so I
knew I had a few minutes before the kids would come storming
down the hallway.

As I sat on the toilet, I had the sense that this was something
more serious than a simple stomach cramp or a bad reaction to
the salad I'd had at lunch. I told Jenny, "I think you better come
in here," which she did—only to catch me a few moments later
when I slumped forward unconscious. If she hadn't been there, I
surely would have fallen and probably would have hit my head
on the tub or, at the very least, crashed onto the tile floor. As it
was, I landed in her arms like a big, limp rag doll. She propped

me back up against the back of the toilet and then I went into a seizure.

That's what she called it, but for a long time I rejected that description, only to see the same term in my medical records when I finally had the courage to look at them years later. It took an equally long time for me to work up the courage to ask her what it looked like, what really happened during the time I was unconscious. My trepidation was well founded. It's an awful scary story, but hearing it and "owning" it has been an important part of my healing.

If the kids had not been just down the hall, she tells me that she would have "screamed her way through it," but as it was, she stayed calm and called out reassuringly to the kids that "Mommy just has an 'owey tummy.' " Knowing she was taking a risk in leaving me, but certain that she had to get to the phone, she said a quick prayer and dashed out to the kitchen. With the receiver in hand, and the kids still (thankfully) engaged in the antics of Baloo and Mogli, she returned to the bathroom, where I was still in full seizure. And as awful as it was, she tells me that what happened next was the scariest of all. Suddenly, the jerking stopped, my muscles relaxed, my skin turned gray, and my temperature dropped like an anchor, leaving me icy cold.

She'd seen a lot already, but now she thought she was watching me die.

When she finally got through to 911, the operator gave her the runaround, quizzing her about whether or not what she'd witnessed was really a seizure. Jenny finally blew her cool, telling the woman she could call it whatever she wanted but she better send an ambulance immediately. Luckily, the fire station is only three minutes away (we'd been there on field trips and for the annual pancake breakfast), and the paramedics arrived while Jenny was still on the phone.

When I came to it was déja vù. The fear and confusion were familiar (although not comforting) and immediately took me back to all the other times I had collapsed. As before, it took me a minute to remember where I was and, as before, fear quickly turned to resolve and resolve into denial.

And that's when I started thinking about mac n' cheese.

I didn't know what had happened but I knew what needed to happen next—everyone needed to calm down and stop panicking. After all, if I went to the hospital who would fix the kids dinner? If there really was something wrong with me, how could I be their mommy? I didn't want to find out and I definitely didn't want to go to the hospital.

Luckily, everyone ignored me. And the next thing I knew, I was being hoisted onto a gurney and rolled out of the house and into the waiting ambulance. By now the kids had abandoned the "electronic baby-sitter" and were watching the whole thing in terror. What happened to mommy? Why is she lying on that funny bed? Why won't those firemen let me talk to her? Where is she going in the ambulance? When will she be back? They had to settle for half answers and halfhearted reassurances because no one really knew what was happening or what would happen next.

At the emergency room I was given two pints of IV fluid and they checked my blood pressure and ran an EKG. Although the tests didn't reveal anything alarming, the ER doc said I should see my physician within twenty-four hours and have him, among other things, recommend a cardiologist. At the time, this barely registered and I have since learned that this is a fairly routine suggestion made to ER patients with fainting symptoms.

But routine or not, they turned out to be the prophetic words of a much-needed guardian angel.

During the weeks that followed my collapse, I underwent more than a half dozen tests to determine the cause of these spells. Each test was scary twice. First, it was scary to schedule and show up for the test. Then, there was the pins-and-needles waiting for the results. It was also exhausting and confusing, as I battled internally with my long-held belief that there was nothing wrong. As each test came back negative, Justus and I were alternately relieved and further confused. At one point they thought I had epilepsy. Then, about ten days later, the neurologist called back to say that, upon further review of my case, the diagnosis was wrong. I was thrilled. I called Justus with great excitement about the news, and got silence on the other end. Sure, he was glad I didn't have epilepsy, but he reminded me, "We still don't know why you've been passing out all these times." Good point, but not one I wanted to hear.

It was hard to know how to feel. While I certainly didn't want to have epilepsy, there had been some comfort in finally having a diagnosis. It was like finding a missing puzzle piece, one that had been missing for years. The diagnosis, I realized, had also held the promise of giving me a chance to dramatically change my life. After all, if a doctor found and pronounced that I really was sick, maybe I'd be forced to take it easy and reprioritize my hectic life. I sensed even then that I couldn't do it on my own. But it might be possible if I was under "doctor's orders" to slow down.

On the other hand, being busy, accomplished, and ambitious had brought me many good things, like promotions, pay raises, and a satisfying career. With the brief period of certainty about my condition over and a return to the diagnostic witch-hunt, I was scared and confused, but I lacked the courage to do anything differently.

During the six weeks between my trip to the ER and my eventual diagnosis, I kept up my Supermom schedule and the pressure on myself to perform, as if to say to myself and everyone else, "See, I'm not sick." My mother would come to town to go with me to the doctor, and then I would ask her to baby-sit so I could work late. I'd schedule my doctor appointments around my meetings, and not the other way around. I'd stop to have my blood drawn on the way home from work. At one point, I was told not to drive, so I learned the bus schedule and took the kids all over town on mass transit.

Never did it occur to me to take a day off, ask my boss if someone else could make the speech, or tell the kids that mommy needed to rest. The nanny kept coming. I kept packing the lunches. The kids went off to school. Full speed ahead.

After epilepsy was ruled out, I went back to see my internist, a friend with whom I had collaborated on some projects at work. Justus and I barged into his office while he was dictating something into his recorder and I started to cry. I said that I wanted to be happy about the epilepsy news but was still scared and confused. He gave me a reassuring hug and suggested it was time for the "tilt-table" test, which we scheduled for five days hence.

With this test, performed in the hospital by a cardiologist, you're strapped to a table and connected to a number of diagnostic machines. The table literally tilts and the machines measure whether your heart is able to get the blood and oxygen where it needs to go regardless of how your body is positioned. It's like an exaggerated form of standing up too fast and getting lightheaded as your body tries to rush blood to your head. Well, this was more than my heart could handle—and it stopped altogether.

My instructions before the test were that I should remain calm and quiet and only speak if I started to "feel anything funny." The table was positioned horizontally like an exam table for the first thirty minutes and then tilted ninety degrees so I was upright, as if standing. This was how things would be for the next forty minutes, or so we thought. The nurses calmly assured me that the thick, eight-inch Velcro straps would keep me from falling "should anything happen." After only seven minutes upright on the table, my heart quit. My file shows that, among other things, I had a grand mal seizure (Jenny was right after all) and the doctor used CPR and mouth-to-mouth to resuscitate me.

After reviving me, Dr. Jackson, my visibly shaken thirty-five-year-veteran cardiologist, announced that what had happened was terrible and need never happen again. What I needed, he said, was a pacemaker.

He could have been speaking a foreign language and I would have understood him better. "What?" I thought. "A pacemaker? Aren't those for old, sick people? Have you noticed that I am not old, that I am not sick, that I am just fine?" I'd even left my suit pants on, thinking that would speed my exit and help me make it to my lunch meeting on time. But this time my protestations didn't ring true. Even though I still had half of my busy-working-mom uniform on, it was clear that I wasn't going anywhere and that mine was a problem that could no longer be ignored.

Later that day when Dr. Jackson's colleague (and the man who would perform my surgery), Dr. Goldreyer, came by to discuss my case, my denial was finally beaten into submission. He showed me the printout from my EKG that morning. Where there was supposed to be a lovely set of peaks and valleys, the visual depiction of a healthy heartbeat, there was nothing but a flat line—the unmistakable portrait of a heart that's stopped. That was the beginning of the end for life, and motherhood, as I knew it. For, just like an alcoholic, drug addict, or gambler, the first step to recovery is admitting that you need help, and I clearly did.

◦   ◦   ◦

The help would come in two forms—and on two different timetables. The physical healing went pretty quickly. Within twenty-four hours, I would have a pacemaker, within forty-eight hours I'd be home from the hospital, and within six weeks I would be "good as new" according to my cardiologist. The emotional healing was another story.

It would clearly take some time, as I didn't immediately acknowledge feeling any of these things. It just wasn't "mommylike." No, the mommylike thing to do (or so I thought) was to get up, brush off, and keep going.

And so four days later I was meeting my boss for lunch to go over what had been happening at the office in my absence. Seven days later I was back at my desk. Nine days after surgery, I was chaperoning the preschool field trip to the pumpkin patch decked out in a purple-and-black satin jester costume complete with boots and pointy hat. By Thanksgiving we were planning to host the family gathering, and by January 1 was preparing for my first postsurgery business trip.

And the whole time, I went on packing lunches, folding the kids' tiny laundry, and rejecting any outside counsel—or personal intuition—suggesting that I may have missed something big.

Like a chance to reexamine the life I had almost lost.

Most of us have an attachment to the activities of our lives. We feel in some way measured by our level of activity and see ourselves as more important when we have more to do. Simplicity is knowing we are enough just the way we are.
—Michelle Morris-Spieker, *The Cherished Self*

How This Book Can Help Sick Moms

Being a sick mom is an experience unlike any other. In the same way that you can't really fathom how dramatically your life will change the moment you give birth to your first child, it's impossible to prepare for the sea change that occurs when you become seriously ill. Of course, this transformation applies to *anyone* who is struck with an illness, but is even more pronounced if you're a mom. That's because moms are givers and sick people must be takers. That's because moms are used to getting things done and handling whatever comes up, and sick people live in a world turned upside down by the unknown and where many days it's a victory simply to take a shower and remember your medicine.

This book arose out of my experience of suffering and recovering from near-fatal cardiac arrest as a thirty-five-year-old mother of two. It is a labor of love whose goal is to show sick moms (and then maybe all moms) that motherhood is not a door through which we pass, leaving all our own needs and desires on the other side. Instead, motherhood can be both a time of self-discovery and self-care even while it is a time of nurturing, giving, and caring for the next generation. And because sick moms are, by definition, unable to carry on as usual, they have a unique opportunity to break these unhealthy, self-sacrificing habits.

More than anything, I hope to show you that life—*your* life—is a series of options, not obligations. If you've had a rigid sense of what moms do and how they act, getting sick gives you an opportunity to change the rules and, possibly, change the answers to questions as simple as "What's for dinner?" and as complex as "How do I balance work and family?"

When you're sick and find that you can't meet all your obligations, you discover you weren't actually *obligated* to do most of them anyway. Those assignments and all those to-dos on your list were merely the by-product of choices you'd made about how and where to spend your time, talent, and energy.

In my case, was there anything wrong with meeting my boss for lunch days after leaving the hospital? Was it a big mistake to chaperon the Halloween field trip or host Thanksgiving dinner? No. The problem is that I didn't consciously choose to do any of these things. I simply felt *obliged* to keep all my previously made commitments and didn't see that I had a choice—even though I had almost died.

Cereal for Dinner is divided into five parts that address how your illness affects you, your kids, your relationships, and your future. In addition to my story and insights, it features anecdotes and loving advice from eighteen other moms, with conditions ranging from cancer to fibromyalgia, from diabetes to heart disease. The insights are neither medical nor "professional," and are not meant to take the place of either. What the book is full of, however, is real, mom-based advice from women who've been there and believe they have something to share. Finally, because sick moms have little time and lots of questions, *Cereal for Dinner* includes lots of lists, suggested activities, resources, and even a few recipes. All this is an effort to remind you that you're not alone, you do have choices, and your illness is merely another chapter in the rich, full story of your life.

Meet the Mommies

As I began work on this book and started to tell friends and family about the project, it quickly became apparent that I had something big on my hands. Whenever I described the book's mission, the listener would invariably relay that he or she knew someone who could use the book—a sister, neighbor, friend, or co-worker. Many also went on to say that they bet this mommy might want to participate in the telling of this story. From these informal conversations grew an informal network of "experts." The only qualifications they needed were that they were or had been sick (with something more than a common cold) and that they had kids. The women you'll be introduced to below, and get to know throughout the pages of this book, have battled cancer, heart disease, diabetes, multiple sclerosis, broken bones, dramatic complications from surgery, and a host of other conditions. Some have recovered, some live with chronic pain. Some spend time in the hospital, some manage their disease from home. Some of them can speak about their condition in the past tense. For others, the present is a struggle and the future is a constant worry.

But all of them understand the struggle of caring for themselves while trying to care for their families. All of them believed their experience could help others and shared freely to make it so. It is with honor and deep gratitude that I introduce them to you now.

Andrea—Spent one year recovering from back surgery and various complications; mom to Madeleine and Kyle.

Catherine—Living with type 1 diabetes; mom to Dylan and Gavin.

Cathy—Ongoing battle with cancer; mother to one daughter.

Darcy—Diagnosed and living with diabetes; mother of Aubrey and Madison.

Fern—Battling cervical cancer; mother of Scott, Dana, Elise, and Iris.

Grace— Living with multiple sclerosis; mom to Andrew and William.

Jackie—Ongoing battle with bilateral optic neuritis, which has resulted in temporary blindness and reduced mobility; mother of Kelsey and Ben.

Jacqueline—Had hysterectomy and mastectomy within one month of each other as doctors discovered a fibroid in her uterus and a malignant lump in her breast; mom to Erin, Brian, and Maya.

Jennie—Breast cancer survivor; mother to daughters Carlyn and Emily.

Jennifer—Battling breast cancer; mother of Alyssa and Bianca.

Marty—Survived two bouts of thyroid cancer; mom to Jimmy, Lisa, Scott, and Alison.

Mary Ellen—Battled multiple cancers for more than two decades; mother of Kristal, Teresa, Stacey, Johnny, and Melissa.

Melissa—Diagnosed and living with multiple sclerosis since she was fifteen years old; Gabriella and Maya's mommy.

Nancy—Suffered pulmonary embolism, pneumonia, and related complications; mom to Meg and Wilson.

Paula—Benign tumor removed from uterus; mother to Alexandra.

Shelley—Diagnosed with gestational diabetes while pregnant with oldest child and continuing to live with the disease; mother to Ben and Taylor.

Stephanie—Two-time cancer survivor and currently living with severe fibromyalgia; mother of Allie.

Sue—Fell down flight of stairs and broke bones in her right leg and left foot and spent twelve months recovering from the breaks and related surgeries and complications; mother of Ryan.

PART I

. . . .

HOW YOUR
ILLNESS AFFECTS YOU

SHOCK

Adjusting to the News
that You're Sick

◉ ◉ ◉ ◉ ◉ ◉ ◉ ◉ ◉ ◉ ◉ ◉ ◉ ◉ ◉ ◉ ◉

We've all heard the numbers—one in eight women will be diagnosed with breast cancer, heart disease is the number-one killer of women in the U.S., and 75 percent of individuals who contract multiple sclerosis are women. And while you may have heard the news, written the checks, and participated in the walk-a-thons, nothing can prepare you for the shock of actually becoming one of these statistics. This is especially true when you're a mother and in the prime of your taking-care-of-everyone-else years.

You're so busy getting everything and everyone to the table you rarely get to eat before your food is stone cold. Your only time alone is when you're on your way to work. You can't even sit on the toilet or take a shower without being interrupted.

This is a mother's world.

That is, until a doctor tells you that you've got a serious, debilitating, or potentially fatal condition, and you need to start thinking about yourself and your health full-time. Not only are you scared, you literally can't see how this is going to work. How will things possibly go on without you at their center, keeping it all together?

You're so concerned about everyone else that you hardly have time to be frightened, at least at first. You ask, "Who's going to take care of the kids?" before you consider "Who's going to take care of me?" You think *we'll see* when the doctor suggests a series of tests and appointments, and wonder who'll drive car pool and address the Christmas cards.

That's what it means to be a mom.

Whether we've been sick for years or are confronted with a sudden health crisis, whether the diagnosis comes quickly or after prolonged testing, we move almost immediately from grappling with what the illness means for *us* to worrying about how our illness is going to impact and inconvenience others.

I can't get sick, everyone is counting on me, we tell ourselves. Although what we need to realize is that now "everyone" is counting on us for something entirely new—they're counting on us to take care of ourselves.

◉ ◉ ◉ ◉ ◉ ◉ ◉ ◉ ◉ ◉ ◉ ◉ ◉ ◉ ◉ ◉

While my first conscious thought after collapsing in the bathroom was about making dinner, when it happened again six weeks later, the first thing on my mind was exercise.

I had just been resuscitated after my "strikingly positive" tilt-table test and my cardiologist was explaining that my very serious condition could be taken care of by implanting a pacemaker to help regulate my heartbeat. As he began to talk about my sympathetic and parasympathetic nervous systems, I had only one burning question, which I blurted out.

"Can I still run?" I queried. Running was something

I'd been doing since joining the track club in eighth grade.

"Yes," he replied. "Lots of my patients with pacemakers jog and even run 10Ks."

Thank God! I thought to myself. And it wasn't so much that I needed to run—I simply need to *know.* And when he answered in the affirmative it was like a promise—a promise that my life with a pacemaker would bear some resemblance to my life before.

⊚   ⊚   ⊚   ⊚   ⊚   ⊚   ⊚   ⊚   ⊚   ⊚   ⊚   ⊚   ⊚   ⊚   ⊚   ⊚   ⊚

In our culture, "sick" means weak, dependent, and needing to take care of *oneself.* "Mom," on the other hand, is synonymous with strong, independent, and taking care of *everyone else.* Sick people are all about tests, doctors' appointments, MRIs, and missed days at work. The two have nothing in common. In fact, it seems to us that they can't coexist.

But the fact is, moms *do* get sick, moms like you and me, and society has given us few tools to deal with the dichotomy of this situation.

So we have to come up with a few of our own.

⊚   ⊚   ⊚   ⊚   ⊚   ⊚   ⊚   ⊚   ⊚   ⊚   ⊚   ⊚   ⊚   ⊚   ⊚   ⊚   ⊚

What to Do Right Now

⊚ Understand that **"sick mom" is not an oxymoron**. You *can* take care of yourself (you have to) and still care for others, but to do so, you must learn to recognize your needs and know when to put them first.

⊚ **Remember the directive given by flight attendants when discussing proper use of oxygen masks in an emergency:** "If you are traveling with a small child, secure your mask before helping with theirs." The point is, if you don't take care of yourself first, you won't be able to take care of them.

◉ **Know that you won't be able to do this alone.** You are going to need shoulders to cry on and people to rely on for everything from rides to the doctor to help with a big project at work. Start thinking about what you need and who can help.

◉ **Swear off guilt** and see that your inability to carry on "as usual" could be the beginning of something new and positive. Really. Everyone (friends, colleagues, even your kids) will be able to adjust to the changes that are inevitable when you get sick. Can you?

◉ ◉ ◉ ◉ ◉ ◉ ◉ ◉ ◉ ◉ ◉ ◉ ◉ ◉ ◉ ◉ ◉ ◉

"Sick Mom" Is Not an Oxymoron

The first thing we have to do is understand that "sick" and "mom" aren't incompatible terms or irreconcilable realities even though it feels that way—especially at first.

The problem is we really have no experience *being* sick. Sure, we've been hit with all the bugs kids bring home from school, but we call that *getting* sick and we rarely let that slow us down. Indeed, it takes something more than a scratchy throat to keep us home from work or looking for someone else to pick the kids up from school. *Getting* sick is about bad luck, *being* sick is about choices.

Being sick means letting yourself miss a deadline, go to the doctor, and maybe even take a nap. *Being* sick means being unreliable or even unavailable. And this, we moms seem to think, may cause the earth to stop turning—or at the very least, homework assignments will be missed, beds will go unmade, and there'll be hell to pay at the office.

So don't be surprised when you find this adjustment difficult. This is all new stuff. For some of us it may be as hard as grappling with the news of the illness itself. So much of our self-definition may be wrapped up in our unmatched ability to do lots of things for lots of people, when we're forced to cut back or slow down, it shakes our very sense of who we are. Paula Spencer, a columnist who writes the "Mom Next Door" column in *Woman's Day* and is a contributing editor at *Parenting* and *Baby Talk*, had this to say in her November 2002 *Woman's Day* column entitled "Mommy Fatigue":

> *I see too many mothers—good mothers—who put everybody else first, always. They have no interests that are not child-related. They claim they have no time to take care of their bodies . . . They confuse selfless mothering with good mothering. Motherhood is not supposed to be so all-consuming that it chews a woman up and spits her out dull, soft, empty and exhausted.*

❖ Mothers' Wisdom ❖

What you learn when you get sick is that even mommies don't get any guarantees. You probably knew that, but in the back of your mind thought, *If anybody deserves a guarantee they're going to be okay it's a mommy,* but mommies get sick just like anybody else.
—Jennifer

When I was first diagnosed with cancer, my immediate thought was *No, I'm not going to have cancer, I am not going to die.* My first thought was *No way, my kids aren't through with me yet.*—Mary Ellen

After my accident, I basically lost a year out of my life. I was in bed for months. I had a live-in housekeeper cleaning my house, cooking in my kitchen, and driving my son wherever he needed to go. She even slept in the guest bedroom upstairs while I was in a rented hospital bed downstairs. Talk about feeling bored, useless, and unmotherly.—Sue

I was very aware from the beginning of the huge logistical turmoil caused by my back surgery. I was in terrible physical pain, but as soon as that subsided, and even sometimes in spite of the pain, I was in emotional turmoil because all I could think about was that I was unable to do all my normal stuff, the stuff everyone counted on me for.—Andrea

I had a hysterectomy and three weeks later found out I had breast cancer. Yes, you can say I was shocked, but I didn't dwell on that long. There was so much to do, to figure out, both about my health and who was going to watch the kids while all this was going on. You couldn't stay in panic or shock for very long because certain things just had to keep happening regardless of what was going on with me.
—Jacqueline

Because our lives as mothers are so full of *doing*—doing the laundry, doing the dishes, doing the right thing—we come to think of ourselves as a collection of activities and accomplishments rather than an individual who needs to be nurtured just as much as we need to nurture.

Oxygen Mask

The folks at the FAA must have had mothers in mind when they drafted the directive that instructs adults to secure their own mask before that of their kids in the case of an emergency. While our instincts when flying on a distressed airplane might be to grab the mask and put it first on our child, there's a chance that would take too long and then we would be at great risk and potentially no help to anyone on the plane, including our child. But while it's common sense, it contradicts a mother's instincts about how to react. Could we really do as instructed when push came to shove? Can we do this when our health is at stake?

Many less serious analogies teach this same lesson. Would you set an empty pitcher before a group of thirsty kids on a summer day? Would you begin a long road trip with your tank on empty? Of course not. Your pitcher and your gas tank would be full. Well, how full is your pitcher? How much is in your tank? Mothering requires a constant exertion of energy and emotion, but we often forget to rest and replenish. And when we're sick, this is serious business.

When dealing with health and sickness, life and death, it's more than just a figure of speech that you can't take care of others if you're not taking care of yourself. For in matters of health, conditions left untreated typically worsen. Whether it's ignoring a scratchy throat and pushing ahead with an overscheduled weekend, or rescheduling your mammogram because your daughter's teacher has asked you to decorate the classroom for Valentine's Day, mothers ignore the small signals, warning signs, and preventive measures at their own peril.

◎　◎　◎　◎　◎　◎　◎　◎　◎　◎　◎　◎　◎　◎　◎　◎　◎

Here, the heart can be a great teacher.

Did you know that before the heart pumps blood anywhere else, even the brain, it feeds itself? It's as if the heart 'knows' that it won't be able to take care of the rest of the body if it doesn't first take care of itself.

As the "heart" and center of most families, moms would do well to do the same.

◎　◎　◎　◎　◎　◎　◎　◎　◎　◎　◎　◎　◎　◎　◎　◎　◎

◆ *Mothers' Wisdom* ◆

Gabriella knows she sometimes has to wait for mommy if she wakes up early and I am too tired to get up yet. She also knows that I can't run about getting her breakfast together until I give myself my shot. Sometimes she has to wait for me—not something three-year-olds are always good at—but she is learning that it's not something mommy can ignore.
—Melissa

It sounds so funny to admit it to someone else, someone who doesn't live with diabetes like I do, but sometimes I have to take food from my kids or have the only granola bar if there's just one left and I know I need to get something to eat quick. Now that they're older, they understand. I'm usually prepared, but they know that if I ask, it's serious.—Darcy

These lessons came the hard way for me. Again and again, first as a young grad student, then a newly married career woman, and then, finally, as a dozen-balls-in-the-air working mother of two, I collapsed, "recovered," and went on as if nothing had happened.

So while I was thinking that I was doing what everyone needed me to do—that is, earning a paycheck, volunteering at school, getting dinner on the table—I was ignoring the only thing that would end up really mattering: my health.

If Jenny hadn't been there to call 911 and set into motion the process that eventually diagnosed and treated my condition, I might not be here. And while *anyone* can go to work, help out in the classroom, or shop for linens for the dorm room, no one can love my kids like I do. Thinking I was helping them grow, I might not have lived to see them grow up.

This is a central lesson that other moms learned as well and shared with me when we spoke.

❧ *Mothers' Wisdom* ❧

I had an interesting experience when I came home from the hospital. I couldn't walk. I had to sit on the couch for pretty much three weeks, and I remember very clearly sitting there watching my family life happen as if it was someone else's family. The dinner and the table-setting and the chores and whose job it is and who gets the backpack down and the homework folder, all that stuff happened without me. And then I realized they don't need me for that stuff. It was a big epiphany for me that for lots of this stuff, anybody can do it—but what anybody can't do is love them and teach them what I want to teach them and convey the values that I want to convey. I was stressing over the stuff that anybody can do.—Jennie

You Won't Be Able to Do This Alone

Once you've recognized that the important distinction between what *you* need to do from what can be easily done by others, you're on your way to getting help and feeling better. The fact is, if you try to do this alone, you'll slow down your healing. It's as simple as that. If you've struggled with being Superwoman or Supermom, maybe you can use your illness as an excuse to bid her farewell.

The oft-quoted adage that "it takes a village" definitely applies here. In our scattered and hectic lives, we don't often feel the sense of community that was so readily available when society moved at a slower pace. Getting sick puts the brakes on, or at least lets us downshift for a while. And in that slowing down, community reappears, connections are made, and help arrives on your doorstep.

We'll talk more later about figuring out what you need and how to ask for it. But I promise that you're already surrounded by all the help you need. Your only job is to ask for it and get out of the way so it can materialize.

❖ *Mothers' Wisdom* ❖

I found that my friends from all the different parts of my life—college, work, the kids' schools, dog-walking friends, neighborhood friends, you name it—they all found each other without me doing anything. They'd all talked and put together a plan to help me before they even knew who was who.—Cathy

When people heard what had happened, they just started coming out of the woodwork, people I knew, people I didn't know, doing all kinds of things for me. It was amazing. —Andrea

The help, asking people for it and receiving it—that's something I swore I would never forget. Asking for help is hard, but you have to do it.—Marty

When I got sick, I had a full-time job caring for my daughter, taking care of the house, everything that goes with that. Suddenly, those became my part-time jobs and getting better was my full-time job. I needed other people to help me with everything else.—Paula

What About the Kids?

I know your kids are never far from your mind and even while you're open to all this good take-care-of-yourself advice, you really want to know what you're going to do about the kids. I understand. Part II of this book is all about that, but let me make one critical point here. The most important thing you can do for your kids is to be good to yourself and honest with them. Think about what they need to know, what they can understand, and then think about how they may respond. They are going to be worried about your health and, depending on your illness, wondering "Are you going to die?" And once you've handled the most emotional topics, they're going to want to know who's going to pick them up from school when you're at the doctor, how long they're going to have to stay there, and what will be for dinner when they get home. Sound familiar? You're going to need love, wisdom, and courage for the first part, and your cadre of helpers for the second.

Good-bye Guilt

Catholic and Jewish comedians joke a lot about growing up in a culture of guilt, but as a group I don't think anyone is more guilt-ridden than moms. We try to do it all and when we can't we feel bad. We're first-rate caretakers but we rarely give ourselves the same care we bestow on others. When we have to slow down, cancel commitments, and upset the family's routine because we're sick, we feel awful. This has to stop. You might have to miss an important deadline at work. Your son might have to play with his less-than-favorite friend after school. Everyone will have to eat the meatless lasagna the church ladies brought over even though it doesn't look like the stuff you make. And your job is to *not worry about it.*

Trust that your kids will adjust and your friends will be glad to help in any way they can. Nip the guilt in the bud because your job is to stop worrying about them and start thinking about what you need to do to get better both physically and emotionally.

❧ *Mothers' Wisdom* ❧

My illness was very hard on my family, but not for the reasons you'd expect. It was hard because of my guilt. It's plain and simple. Now that it's over I see how silly that was. I wish I'd known what to do with those feelings.—Sue

It's amazing how guilty you can feel. You have to go to the doctor, take naps, take your medicine, manage your energy, but that doesn't mean your mind isn't running around wildly thinking about all the other things you "should" or "would" be doing, all the things "normal" moms do.—Stephanie

I do not honestly know how to accept so much from so many.—Cathy

THREE TENNIS BALLS AND A FLAMING SWORD

What It Feels Like to Juggle Illness and Motherhood

◦ ◦ ◦ ◦ ◦ ◦ ◦ ◦ ◦ ◦ ◦ ◦ ◦ ◦ ◦ ◦ ◦ ◦ ◦

After getting over the shock of discovering that you're sick (well, you never *really* get over the shock but you wrestle it into a box so you can get through each day), you may start looking at your illness as a project.

Like finding a kindergarten for your five-year-old or a nursing home for your aged parent, you can do this stuff with your eyes closed. Mothers are proficient multitaskers. We're pros at dissecting the task, doing the research, and getting the information needed to make a good decision—all the while keeping all our other balls in the air.

The problem is, this project is all about us—and it doesn't lend itself to being juggled. This "project" shakes our sense of who we are. It demands of us new skills and stirs up our emotions. And if your illness is one in which death is even a remote possibility the consequences are staggering.

❖ *Mothers' Wisdom* ❖

Everyone knows that being a mom is all about juggling, keeping all your balls in the air, but finding out you have cancer or some other life-threatening condition is like being tossed a flaming sword and being asked to juggle that too in addition to the three tennis balls you're already trying to keep airborne. None of the other stuff goes away, but now one of the things you're juggling could kill you.—Jennifer

The fact is, the standard run-of-the-mill juggling that we've become so proficient at as a mother might actually hurt us in this situation. Just because we *can* do a million things at once, *should we?* The reality of being a sick mom is, more than anything else, a reality of less and not more. Less time, less energy, less patience, less everything. So, it would naturally follow, we should pare back our to-do list to its bare essentials. To keep Jennifer's analogy alive, we might have to drop a few of the tennis balls (e.g., the inconsequential things) in order to keep the flaming sword safely in flight. Because, after all, the sword is the only one that can kill us.

CHECKUP FROM THE NECK UP

The Emotional Aspects
of a Physical Illness

* * * * * * * * * * * * * * * * * * *

About six weeks after my surgery, my doctor ecstatically proclaimed that I was "all better" and that I could go back to all my usual routines and activities. "I release you with no restrictions" were his exact words. While there truly was much to celebrate, I soon discovered that my heart problem had been replaced by a "head problem." We'd answered the medical question, but so many others still remained. What was I supposed to do now? Who was going to help me deal with the trauma and confusion that accompanied my physical collapse? Am I still the same person I was before or someone new entirely? Sure, my heart was beating again, but it still ached. Who would help me with that?

* * *

When you're a sick mom, it's often all you can do to get to the doctor, remember to take your medicine, and rearrange your schedule so you can go to physical therapy. The last thing you want someone to suggest is that there's something else you need to do, another appointment you need to make. But there is. I strongly encourage you to see a therapist; because my experience is that this stuff is just too big to handle alone. Professional counselors provide a safe place to talk about how scary it is to contemplate death at an early age and imagine your kids growing up without you. They serve as nonjudgmental sounding boards who'll listen to you complain that your husband isn't helping enough or that your kids are driving you crazy. The good ones listen well. The best ones also provide perspective and sage advice.

◉ ◉ ◉ ◉ ◉ ◉ ◉ ◉ ◉ ◉ ◉ ◉ ◉ ◉ ◉ ◉ ◉

There has been a positive trend in recent years with more and more employers providing at least some mental health coverage as part of a package of benefits. Such policies typically allow for a finite number of visits before the patient has to pick up most or all of the cost. Check your policy for coverage details or talk to the HR department at work (some larger companies even offer in-house counseling through an employee assistance program). If you don't have coverage for such benefits, you might try free or low-cost group programs offered through local nonprofits, hospitals, or associations (Multiple Sclerosis Society, American Diabetes Association, etc.).

◉ ◉ ◉ ◉ ◉ ◉ ◉ ◉ ◉ ◉ ◉ ◉ ◉ ◉ ◉ ◉ ◉

I learned the hard way how crucial it is that you not underestimate the emotional toll of your illness, and a good psychologist can help with that. Healing your psyche might take longer than healing your body. For while doctors and nurses draw blood, study charts, and look for a cure, they aren't overly concerned with how you're feeling emotionally. It's not that they don't care; it's just that it's not their job.

So you have to make it *your* job.

If the idea of talking to a professional is too scary to contemplate at first, start with your partner, sister, mother, or close friend. Find somebody who you can totally confide in, someone who *won't* try to convince you that "It's all going to be okay" when that's not how you're feeling, someone who won't say "Don't worry" when worry is all you can do.

You might also try a support group where you can share in a setting where the people listening aren't emotionally involved with your illness but are understanding and supportive. Support groups can be found through the local chapters of all the major disease associations, through local hospitals and community groups, and by searching on-line.

When you begin, some of your feelings are going to be right on the surface, easy to access, and some are going to come up after a lot of digging. For some people, illness reminds them of other losses they've suffered throughout life or triggers memories and anxieties connected with being sick as a child.

This was my experience. Through my work with a therapist, I was eventually able to identify that my resistance to seeking medical attention all those years (and the ferocity of my denial while we were trying to figure out what was wrong) was due in some part to fear and negative feelings associated with illness, doctors, and hospitals from my earliest days. Indeed, as a four-pound preemie not allowed to go home with her mother until three weeks after delivery, I got a sense early on that the hospital was a lousy place and that being sick was a lousy proposition.

No matter what your previous health history or experience with doctors and hospitals, getting sick when you're a mother shakes up the bedrock assumptions you have about your role in the lives of the people around you and, in so doing, sends your self-image on a panicked trek to discover whether you're still the same you. And the answer is both yes and no.

❧ *Mothers' Wisdom* ❧

I used to clean the house, now I have a maid. I used to cook the dinner, now my neighbors bring it over. I used to be the one who picked my kids up from school and was with them all afternoon, now friends and baby-sitters do that. I even lost my hair and my breasts, my femininity. So, I ask you, who am I now? Sometimes I look in the mirror and I see myself. Sometimes I look and I don't know who that is.—Jennifer

It took me many months to understand what a shock my illness had dealt to my self-image. But when I did, my healing truly began—and I couldn't have done it without some help.

❉   ❉   ❉

Given the valuable insights and boost in self-esteem I've gained from therapy in the aftermath of my illness, I was surprised at how few of the moms I talked to while working on this book had sought any help from a therapist or counselor. I think reaching out for this kind of help was one of the few areas where I really did take care of myself. Whether it's dealing with issues of body image or feeling useless because you can't do all the things you used to do for everyone who's counting on you, it helps to have someone to talk to. I'm not alone in thinking this is a good idea.

Elise NeeDell Babcock, author of *When Life Becomes Precious: The Essential Guide for Patients, Loved Ones and Friends of Those Facing Serious Illness* (Bantam, 2002) and founder of Cancer Counseling, Inc. a first-of-its-kind agency providing free professional counseling to cancer patients and their families, agrees that sick mommies should try therapy—and she thinks the magic number is (at least) three visits. "I think getting this kind of help is crucial, and I always tell people they have to go at least three times before they can decide if they think it's working for them. It takes that long to get comfortable and determine if they've got a 'fit' with the therapist," she says. "And just because you don't like one therapist doesn't mean you're not going to like any therapist. It's worth working at it because this kind of help can be invaluable."

The process can take some time and you might not be ready to start right away. It can also take many forms, from traditional one-on-one counseling to support groups to journaling or seeking help from a trusted advisor, such as a cleric at your place of worship. Regardless, I encourage you not to overlook the emotional aspects of what may seem like an entirely physical ordeal. Because it's so much more than that.

I can say without hesitation that the mental/emotional/spiritual changes in my life since my illness have been tremendous, and, because of them, what was a crisis has become a blessing. I can also say that I wouldn't have been able to get to this place and achieve this level of understanding and peace without professional guidance. Therapy was the cocoon that transformed my fear and uncertainty into understanding, acceptance, and gratitude.

You may or may not find that the same applies to you, but I encourage you to find out.

Where to Look for Help

How to Find a Therapist:

The best way to find a good therapist is through a referral. Ask friends of yours if they know of or have been to someone good. You can also secure a referral from your doctor, local hospital, or the HR department at your company (or your husband's). Like all personnel matters, those conversations will be considered private and confidential. If, however, this still makes you uncomfortable, try cold-calling a few "approved providers" from your insurance directory or your local Yellow Pages and ask a few questions to see if you can find a good fit. Also, remember that it may not be a long-term relationship, and that you may try a few before finding the right person for you.

There's a nice site on the Internet called About Psychotherapy (*www.aboutpsychotherapy.com*). It is hosted by a clinical psychologist and answers questions such as: "What is psychotherapy?" "How does it work?" and "Why go?" It also has a section called "Choosing a Therapist" that helps guide you toward the kind of therapist that might be best for you.

What about Books?

The "self-help" section at the bookstore is one of the biggest and fastest growing. Authors offer tips on life's big questions and provide widely varying approaches to uncovering readers' fears and helping them set new goals. There are journals, thought-a-day calendars, and books on meditation, prayer, and relationships. You name the problem, question, or concern and it's probably been written about. Browse through this section on-line or, if you have the energy, at the corner store or the local library and see what strikes your fancy. A few of my favorites when I was sick and getting better were:

When Bad Things Happen to Good People, by Harold Kushner
The Cherished Self, by Michelle Morris-Spieker
Kitchen Table Wisdom, by Dr. Naomi Remen
When Life Becomes Precious, by Elise Babcock
The Victoria's Secret Catalog Never Stops Coming and Other Lessons I Learned from Breast Cancer, by Jennie Nash

While books, support groups, and therapists can all help and guide you as you explore the meaning of your illness, the real "expert" in all of this is *you*. Don't forget to create a time and a place for self-reflection as the feelings you unearth during this time of crisis may be the very stuff upon which you'll build a more healthy future for you and your family. I find it most helpful to write these feelings down and use a "free-flow" approach where I don't worry about spelling, punctuation, or penmanship. And while I may never read what I've written to another soul— or even again to myself—the process of writing it down always brings the feelings into relief.

✔ TRY THIS

Grab a journal, notebook or some pretty stationery to answer one, some, or all of these questions. (Alternately, you might be in the mood to doodle, start a grocery list, or simply move on. Do what feels right for you, no shoulds, have-tos, or guilt!)

At this moment, the one word that best sums up my feelings about being sick is _____.

I'm trying to keep it together, but if no one were watching I would be _____.

My biggest challenge now is _____.

What nobody seems to understand is _____.

My biggest fear is _____.

When this is all over I am going to _____.

REACHING OUT

How to Ask for Help and Receive What Is Given

⊚　⊚　⊚　⊚　⊚　⊚　⊚　⊚　⊚　⊚　⊚　⊚　⊚　⊚　⊚　⊚

*After the verb "to Love," "to Help" is the
most beautiful verb in the world.*

—BERTHA VON SUTTNER,
　author, activist, Nobel Peace Prize winner, 1905

More dangerous than any ailment or medical emergency, I
believe, is women's inability to ask for help. In my case
and the case of every mother I spoke to for this book, no one asks
because no one wants to be seen as needy.

Again and again, the moms I met said things like "I didn't
want to impose," "They all have their own lives going on," and
"I knew I wouldn't be able to reciprocate" to explain why they
suffered alone through much of their illness rather than reaching
out for help. And these were women with brain tumors, kidney
failure, multiple broken bones, and cancer, women who everyone

would agree "qualified" as being needy and for whom asking for help would have made a lot of sense. Why is it, then, that women, even very sick women, find it so hard to ask for help? I have a few ideas.

In some cases, it's our "good girl" training that insists that our needs be placed at the bottom of the heap so as not to disrupt or trump anyone else's. It's a mind-set that keeps us from asking all the questions we have at the doctor because we don't want to "take too much of his or her time" or keep other patients waiting.

In addition, I think our struggle to ask for help results from the rather boundaryless world in which modern mothers find themselves. Women now have nearly unfettered access to interesting roles in all aspects of society, but we added these new roles without eliminating any of the old ones. As such, women have entered the workforce in droves but still take primary responsibility for the housework, shopping, and childcare duties in most families. So, whether we choose to work outside the home or not, it's assumed that we'll handle whatever comes up on the domestic front. And as Donna Reed, June Cleaver, and Carol Brady didn't need any help (well, Carol did have Alice), we don't feel we have the right to ask for any either.

Finally, on a very basic level, being solely a giver and never a receiver may simply be a bad habit. And at the core of this bad habit, on a very deep level, may be the troubling truth that we don't value ourselves enough.

For so many reasons, this has to change and our illness may provide the perfect opportunity to make that shift.

How to Ask for Help:
A Primer

● You can't be in denial and ask for help at the same time.

● When you get sick, life as you've lived it is suspended. Even if you've never been good at asking for help before, you can start, and no one will be the least surprised.

● Make a list of the things you would like help with.

● Make a separate list of all the people in your life who could help you.

● Start making assignments. If you're rusty and hesitant, set a goal to ask for help with one thing a day until you're ready to ask for more.

● Learning how to ask for help could be one of the most positive and lasting gifts of your illness.

Help and Denial

You don't want to be sick. I'm guessing that you're scared and angry, and you wish it would all just go away. You want your old life back. You've given in to the reality of doctors' appointments, tests, and medicine, but you refuse (for as long as possible) to let it disrupt the rest of your life. You'll squeeze in "the health stuff" so long as you don't have to change too much of the rest. But that's just crazy.

We talked earlier about denial, but it bears repeating here because denial is like a wall that separates you from the assistance you need. It's the dike holding back a huge reservoir of help.

I know.

I was there.

What else but anger and denial could have propelled me to go so frenetically about my routine during the weeks before and after my diagnosis and surgery? I didn't accept my illness so I couldn't ask for help, and it wasn't until I admitted that I was sick that I could truly start to heal.

◉   ◉   ◉

I recently ran into an old friend, the mom of some kids who were in preschool with mine during the time of my illness. While we were talking, the subject of my illness came up, and she said, "I wish I would have known that you were sick and what you needed. We all wondered, but all of a sudden you were back and it was like things were fine, and so no one wanted to say anything because no one knew what happened."

Then, just after that, I was leafing through one of the many journals I had kept at the time, and came across a small coupon book lovingly made for me with construction paper and colored markers by another dear friend. The handmade coupons could have been redeemed for home-cooked meals, kid-free afternoons, and two or three trips to the grocery store. I say, "could have been" because they're all still there. I didn't use a single one.

I can see now that I was so afraid to admit to myself (and to others) that I was sick and that I needed help, that I acted as if everything was fine. And, while deep down I wanted casseroles, car pools, and play dates to appear on my doorstep, my I-can-handle-it performance was so convincing that these things never materialized. One negated the other. So let go of the anger, drop the denial, and let the help and the healing begin.

✔ Try This

Grab your journal or some pretty paper again and consider this question:

I'm sick and I can't take care of everyone and still take care of myself. I need to ask for help and that makes me feel . . .

Let the anger, sadness, and frustration flow onto the page. After you've finished, read it to someone: your therapist, husband, mother, friend—or even out loud to yourself. This small act can have tremendous impact. For once you "own" the anger and the illness, you can get out of your own way and start asking for help.

Even If You've Never Been Good at Asking for Help, You Can Start

One blessing that comes from being sick is that the crisis briefly suspends the norm, the routine, "the way things have always been." And if the status quo finds you ignoring your needs, your illness creates an opening whereby you can try out some new behavior. For getting sick suspends all the rules and people will look to you for clues about how you want to be treated and whether you want to be helped. Everyone's watching, so err on the side of being needy and then turn away the seventeenth turkey-noodle casserole that arrives rather than end up with only one.

In the early stages of any mom's illness, there are going to be moments when it's simply not possible for things to carry on as they always have. The kids may have to go to school with a neighbor, even though you have always driven them. Your husband may have to leave late for work because he's helping with the kids. Your boss may have to ask someone else to develop the marketing plan for the company's new gizmo even though that has long been your forte.

For both you and everyone involved, these are golden moments.

Because you're too sick, tired, or busy with doctor's appointments to meet your regular obligations, others have to step up, pitch in, be flexible and forgiving. And if you're lucky—and smart!—you may be able to start a trend that will be sustained even when you're back on your feet.

On my list of things I'd do differently next time, I would have taken as much medical leave as my employer allowed and my family could afford. I would have reneged on all my volunteer commitments, and I would have lined up a few weeks of home-cooked meals.

❧ *Mothers' Wisdom* ❧

I didn't want to ask anybody for anything, but I didn't have a lot of choice. I couldn't walk, stand, bend, or drive. I have to admit I had a strong resistance to asking for help and the help I got either just showed up from friends who didn't wait to be asked or came because I hired someone to do the work. I was lucky we could afford the help we got because I think I would have been in bad shape if I'd had to rely on my ability to ask for what I needed.—Andrea

I can say without a doubt that encouraging women to ask for help when they're sick is the biggest advice I could give from my experience.—Mary Ellen

If these few examples are any indication, and I think they are, a revolution is needed in how women view help. The problem is not that sick moms don't know how to ask for help; it's that women in general don't know how to ask and that doesn't change when they *do* get sick. We absolutely need to grow as comfortable asking for help as we are with giving it—and getting sick just might get us started.

What Kind of Help Do You Need? Make a List

To help get you started, think of all the things you do in a day, a week, a month. Heck, think of all the things you do before 9:00 A.M. most mornings. If you're like most moms, you are most likely in charge of your children's basic necessities and the details of running your home. Depending on how old your kids are, these responsibilities may look a bit different, but they are your domain nonetheless. (And this seems to be true whether you work outside the home part-time, full-time, or not at all.)

For example, if you've got a toddler, you must bathe and dress her, make her something to eat. If you've got an older child, you have to know if his favorite red NASCAR T-shirt is clean (or clean enough) and are sure to have his favorite lunch meat in the fridge. If it's a teenager you've got, she will need to go shopping for a prom dress, have help with her science project, and she'll want to show you some Web sites for the universities where she's interested in applying next fall. If your son is coming home from college for the holidays, you can bet he's going to arrive with a bag full of laundry and an empty stomach.

You get the picture. Even if you don't have to *do* everything yourself, even if you've got a totally involved dad, independent-minded kids, a housekeeper or a nanny, usually it's mom who knows when it's time to buy peanut butter, shoes, and toothbrushes. It's mom who knows when the gardener comes, when the DVDs have to be returned, and the date Johnny's due home for spring break.

So, what happens when mom can't? In an upcoming chapter,

we'll talk about serving cereal for dinner (and pizza, leftovers, and KFC) and other shortcuts that facilitate healing, but in this chapter, we're doing something even more critical—dissecting and debunking the myth that tells women, and especially moms, that they have to do everything for everyone even when this puts them at risk. Not every mom falls victim to this fiction, but it's all around us as TV, movie, and magazine moms expertly juggle myriad needs at work, home, and elsewhere and never look the worse for it. But that isn't reality. Whether we're Supermom or supertired mom, we all can use a little help—especially when we're sick.

✔ TRY THIS

So let's make a list of things you need help with. I say anything that keeps you from taking a nap or makes you late for a doctor's appointment needs to be written down (or recited to a friend who's offered to help). Anything that causes you stress or makes you tired goes on the list. Here are a few examples:

- laundry
- grocery shopping
- dusting
- making lunches
- cooking dinner
- picking up dry cleaning
- watering the yard
- getting an oil change

- paying the bills

- keeping the kids entertained

- taking the dog to the vet

- preparing for a meeting at work

- checking e-mail

- returning phone calls

You can make one long list or break it down by day (e.g., Monday, take Sarah to band practice; Wednesday, call James about upcoming marketing presentation; Friday: send in fee for Michael's drama camp) or by category (e.g., work, children, pet, house, spouse, etc.) It's basically the to-do list you know so well *but this time you're going to give it away.*

Go through the list and move to the bottom anything that can wait at least two weeks, and eliminate anything that can be skipped altogether. Then, look at the remaining list and put an asterisk next to anything that you absolutely have to do yourself (this list should be short). What's left is what you need to delegate.

Before we start making assignments, I want to say one thing about the short list of things you keep for yourself to do. In speaking to moms for this project and analyzing my own actions and decisions while sick, I learned that you can't go from doing *everything for everyone* to doing *nothing for anyone.* It's too big a change. It's not possible, nor is it recommended. Sick moms need to stay involved and engaged. It's good for their psyches. But they have to make choices and cut back. You're going to want to know who's picking up your kids, but you may not have to be the one to set it up. You may want to spend some time in the kitchen, but maybe all you do is make the salad to go with the pasta your neighbor brought over. You may take a call from a colleague at work to help her prepare for an upcoming meeting, but you don't need to attend the meeting—or even listen in via speakerphone.

The beauty of learning how to ask for help is that we decide what matters most and what's most realistic given our circumstances, and we shed the rest. This is different from our usual modus operandi where there's often little conscious choice about what goes on the list and we simply "do until we drop" each day.

❖ *Mothers' Wisdom* ❖

As a mom, you're wired to be the primary caretaker. You may have just learned that you're going to lose your breast or you may be so drugged with narcotics that the room spins, but somehow, you're still thinking about your kids. You're still planning what they're going to eat for dinner, worrying about whether they got their homework done, wondering who's going to drive them to school, and whether or not you've given them the tools to understand sex, God, and global warming. You want to start thinking more about yourself, but find it's near impossible.—Jennie

Who Can Help?
Make a List

When meeting facilitators are trying to help a group reach consensus about how to solve a thorny issue at work or spur creative thinking about a long-standing challenge, they often plaster the conference room walls with butcher paper and encourage everyone to shout out any and all ideas they've got. The admonition to all is that ideas should be shared without self-censorship and received without judgment. In this model, every idea is a good one and there are no wrong answers.

If you're having trouble making a list of things you'd like help on or are hesitant to start making a list of who might help, keep this strategy in mind. You may even go as far as having your husband bring home some paper or posterboard from the office, or simply use some scratch paper you have lying around the house. The point is you want to think *big* when you start. And remember, no one has to see these lists but you, and you don't have to execute on every "outlandish" idea you come up with. You may find however, that asking your mother-in-law to fold your laundry or your neighbor to walk your dog is not as crazy as you think.

✔ TRY THIS

Start by thinking very broadly about the people in your life who can be of assistance during this trying time. You may not even have to know someone particularly well to enlist his or her help. Some candidates include:

- ◎ your husband

- ◎ your mom

- ◎ your mother-in-law

- ◎ your siblings

- ◎ your neighbors

- ◎ friends (from temple, mosque, yoga class, book club)

- ◎ your kids (with age-appropriate tasks)

- ◎ other parents (from school, the drama club, your child's pottery class, Sunday school, soccer team, etc.)

Start Making Assignments

Now that you've got your list, you have to make your first request. You have to ask someone to help you get the help you need. Seriously. Give your list to a friend, your mother, or partner and ask them to start matching people up with tasks. Provide any information they might need to match the right people with the right task. (e.g., "Marni can pick the kids up from school because she's already picking up her kids and she lives close." Or, "Ask my secretary to call Tom in the marketing department and ask him to handle that presentation.") If you can, direct your helper to your e-mail list, phone book, or the kids' class roster so you don't have to go hunting around for the information. Then, it's hands off. Let your friend make the calls and send the e-mails. Tell your pal you only want updates on a need-to-know basis and remain calm when you don't hear anything for a while.

Some months after my illness, another mom at my kids' pre-school became sick. Her husband brought in a blank calendar and asked people at the school to sign up to make dinners for the family while she was in the hospital and recuperating. It worked beautifully and the warm, delicious meals started appearing.

Recalling this, another mom at the school used this same system when she broke her ankle and couldn't drive her son to school. She asked someone to put together a sign-up sheet and post it at school and we all signed up to take William to and from school until she got the cast off her driving foot.

This all seemed natural and right. It was great to know just what they needed and a joy to be able to provide it—but first they had to ask.

Learning to Ask for Help Could Be the Most Important Gift of Your Illness

When we can't tell people what we need when we're sick, it's because we never practiced this skill when we were well. This has to change. If and when sick mommies do ask for help, they try to keep it to a bare minimum. This has to change as well.

❖ *Mothers' Wisdom* ❖

I had asked a friend to take me to my initial surgeon's visit. It lasted three hours and I cried in pain the whole way home. So, when I had to go to another appointment and my husband couldn't take me, he hired a car and a driver to pick me up and take me there. When my girlfriend found out, she was furious. She said, 'I thought we were friends,' and she was serious. But I just couldn't imagine asking her again after what she'd done before.—Andrea

Without even realizing it, you keep track of who's done what and how often and you keep a mental list of IOUs because when you get better you'll want to pay them back.—Jacqueline

Sometimes I ask my husband to do things around the house like the dishes or clean the bathroom floor, but I usually do it before he gets around to it. I can't just let it go.—Fern

I heard these sentiments again and again as I talked to moms who had been sick, and they were poignant reminders of my own long-standing inability to ask for help.

Here's a small but significant example of how I've begun to live by a new modus operandi, one that includes asking for help. The other day I was picking up my son from a play date, which was itself helpful to me to have him out of the house for a while because Addie had gotten a similar invite and with both of them gone, I saw a chance to rest before beginning the nighttime routine. I'd been feeling under the weather. It was about four o'clock when I pulled up in front of Dylan's house, and I was feeling lousy.

My plan had been to get Travis and then stop at the market on the way home because we needed a few things (Addie was being dropped off later). But as I got out of the car, I realized there was no way I was going to make it to the market. I just wanted to go home, slap together some grilled cheese sandwiches, and get the kids to bed, with me following shortly thereafter. So, what did I do? I asked Dylan's mom, Joanna, if she had an extra bar of soap and roll of toilet paper, which was all I really needed that couldn't wait until the next day. At the time, we hardly even knew each other but Joanna has such a generous spirit I knew practicing my newfound skill on her would not be too risky.

She said yes so naturally, quickly pulling the requested items from the pantry, that I knew it was giving her joy, too. Such a little thing, yet such a big deal, such an opportunity for growth—and all this because I could admit that I felt too crummy to go to the store.

When I had heart surgery, I couldn't ask for a home-cooked meal or a day off from work. Now here I was with just a scratchy throat and I was asking an acquaintance for household sundries. I'd come a long way. You can too.

Remember what Jennifer said earlier about needing energy for the battle? The only one who can battle your disease is you.

Other people can cook.

Other people can clean.

Other people can pick up the kids, the groceries, and the laundry.

If you let other people do some of this stuff, you'll have more energy for your fight—the only thing that really matters.

Everything else will take care of itself. Only you can take care of you.

DINNER ON THE DOORSTEP

A Covered Dish Is Worth a Thousand Floral Bouquets

· · · · · · · · · · · · · · · · · ·

Maybe it's because women are still the primary cooks in most families and because the daily question of "What's for dinner" is as inescapable as a basket of unfolded laundry, but there's nothing quite as wonderful as having something warm and delicious to serve your family—when you didn't have to lift a finger to get it on the table. For years, the casserole was the "gift to give" to a family in need, especially if the *person* in need was the mom. Now it's just as likely to be a Chinese chicken salad or a crock of lentil soup, but the point is the same—and so is the joy in receiving it.

So how is it that I, a woman with a tremendous network of friends, colleagues, and acquaintances, only received one ready-to-eat meal? What kind of breakdown was there in the social fabric of my community that no one thought to put food on our table when I was sick?

The answer? They saw me at the market.

Truly, I was back at the dry cleaners, back buying groceries and acting as though nothing had happened before most of my friends even had time to get out a cookbook or locate their Pyrex. Through both my words and my actions I telegraphed a message to everyone around me that I didn't need any help. And so I didn't get any.

To be honest, there was one casserole, and it is noteworthy because it came from Michelle. Michelle is a friend of a friend. I barely know her, and had I known her better she probably wouldn't have gone to the trouble.

Michelle heard through the grapevine that I was sick, then ran into my mom at the market and asked if she could bring over a meal. My mom graciously accepted on my behalf and it was done. The next day it arrived, chicken, almonds, and French-cut green beans. You know, the kind with the can of Campbell's soup that kind of holds it all together? Nothing fancy, nothing gourmet, but it was warm and delicious. "Comfort food" in every sense of the word and a true gift from the heart.

I just wish I had known to ask for more of it.

◈   ◈   ◈

There are probably as many ways to give and receive help as there are people giving and receiving it. I asked all the moms I interviewed to tell me the nicest thing anyone did for them. Here is some of what they told me, followed by the three things that came to mind when I considered this same question. Take a read. Make a list. Some of this might sound good to you.

◈ Mothers' Wisdom ◈

A mother from my daughter's school, with whom I am only slightly acquainted, organized a whole group of people to make lunches for my daughter for the rest of the school year. Someone even took her to the store and asked her to point out the things she liked to eat and they spread the word. This went on for about a month and a half before I was even aware of it. This was a huge gift to both me and my husband who was trying to manage so many other things.—Cathy

One dear friend brought me apples one day at the hospital when I complained that it was impossible to get good fruit. Another brought me tea and beautiful china cups too, and we had a little tea party right there on my bed. It was a little thing that kept me feeling human. A group of friends who lived too far away to visit or bring casseroles pitched in and got us a gift certificate for a great local caterer. We're still picking up meals from there when we're not up to cooking.—Nancy

One friend started bringing fresh flowers and leaving them on my doorstep once a week. She's still doing that even though my illness is "old news" now and some of the original help has faded away. I still get my flowers and that's her way of saying "I'm still thinking of you" even though I've been sick for a while.—Jennifer

My sister called one day and asked if I needed anything and to my surprise I said yes. I asked her to pick me up some of those Ensure protein drinks. She brought me different flavors and when I told her which one I liked best, she went and got me a whole case.—Mary Ellen

Friends came over and took my dirty laundry home to wash. I protested but they ignored me.—Andrea

There were lots of casseroles, food from people I didn't even know, but the nicest thing anyone did was when I went out to lunch and told one of my friends that I had decided not to have reconstructive surgery (after a double mastectomy) and that a lot of my friends were questioning my decision. She simply said, "Well, why would you want to?" and that gave me the courage to move forward with what felt right to me.—Jacqueline

I needed a ride to the hospital every day for six weeks for treatment. Some ladies from church organized a schedule and took me, waited for me, and drove me home every day for six weeks and afterward thanked me for the "privilege" of helping out. Imagine that.—Jennie.

Three things came to mind when I put this same question to myself.

First was the dedication of my mom, who came up and stayed with us and took care of the kids, cooked for us, and screened my calls and visitors. She created a buffer around me to keep things as calm as possible, which still was not enough to keep me down for long but probably bought me a couple of critical days at the beginning. Second was a friend at work who gave us her cabin in the mountains for a few days (and my boss who encouraged us to go). I was feeling better by that time, just tired, so it was a great chance for all of us to get out of town and have a little fun together. Finally, there was Michelle's casserole, which has come to symbolize my journey in learning to ask for help but was delicious in its own right. (I just hope I remembered to return the Corningware.)

Oh, and that reminds me, ask people to come back and get their pots, pans, and dishes from you, or assign a friend to coordinate all that. Or better yet, ask those bearing gifts of food to use disposable dishes. The last thing you need to be thinking about when you're trying to heal is cleaning and returning your friends' dirty cookware.

Letting Others Help You
Helps Them Too

Although I got only one casserole, I got tons of flowers, cards, and get-well wishes. It was clear from the daisies, roses, and cookie bouquets strewn about the house that I had no lack of friends. I just didn't know how to turn all that love and all those good wishes into help because I didn't know how to ask, and when help was offered I didn't know how to respond.

Stephanie, whose fibromyalgia leaves her not knowing from day to day whether she's going to be able to leave the house or even get out of bed, has had to build an extensive network of helpers after years of illness.

> *When I had cancer, I was lousy at asking for help. I guess I got better at it with this new condition because it quickly became clear that I absolutely had no choice but to ask for and accept help. And what I've discovered in the meantime is how much people want to help. It's really lovely—and it's cruel to turn down help you need from a friend who's offered.*

When I heard this from Stephanie, it reminded me of something I'd learned about the tools and techniques that bring people success in twelve-step programs like Alcoholics Anonymous. Providing service is one of the tools of the program; it's in the literature. The concept is that you solidify your own recovery by giving back to others. Helping others and helping yourself are one and the same.

Soon after, I had the chance to be of service myself.

The couple next door is in their late sixties with kids my age and a big network of family and friends. When they go out of town, they have a friend who feeds the dogs, cuts the grass, and collects the mail. When they need a ride to the airport, their son or daughter steps up. They have so many friends, so many *helpers*, that I often wonder what *I* can do for them in return for all they've done for us (hand-me-down books and toys from their grandkids, letting our dog out if she's whining when we're gone, collecting our mail, taking in our empty trash cans, etc.). So, when I heard that Ann was scheduled for back surgery, I assumed everything would be taken care of and I'd settle for buying her some flowers and a get-well card.

Then a wonderful thing happened. Ann's husband, Kenny, knocked on the door the afternoon before the operation and asked if I could do them a favor.

"Sure, anything," I responded. Getting an actual assignment was even better than trying to guess what kind of flowers she'd like.

"Can you go to the farmer's market tomorrow and pick up Ann's favorite strawberries?" he inquired.

When I enthusiastically agreed, he passed me some money in an envelope ("That should cover it"), discussed with me how I would know which ones were the ripest and the sweetest, and how many to buy ("Usually we get half a tray, but if they look good, get the whole tray") and finally some notes about the exact vendor they like to buy from ("The second booth on the left when you're coming from the parking lot"). And, interestingly, the more complicated it became, the more excited I got because I knew it was important and I would be getting exactly what she wanted and needed.

When I returned the next afternoon with the flat of red juicy fruit, I felt like Santa Claus.

Easy Dinners You Can Make— Or Have A Friend Make for You (No chopping required!)

CROCKPOT CHICKEN

1 one-pound pre-cut chicken
1 jar of salsa

Rinse chicken pieces in cold water and place in Crockpot. Open salsa and pour onto chicken. Cook on LOW for six hours or HIGH for two hours. Serve with rice (instant) and black beans (from a can). You won't believe how good this is! Serves 4 (with some leftovers).

HAM & CHEESE MELTS

2 slices whole wheat bread, toasted
2 slices of Swiss cheese (or your choice)
1 slice cooked ham

Place slice of toast onto paper towel. Top with slice of cheese, slice of ham, and second slice of cheese. Cover with remaining toast. Fold 3 of 4 corners of paper towel toward center, covering like an envelope. Turn and place folded-side down on microwave-safe plate. Cook on HIGH 30 to 45 seconds, until cheese melts. (Tips: Place toast on the diagonal so that the folding is easier. Also, prepare each envelope first and then heat one at a time and everyone can sit down together.) Each "envelope" makes one sandwich.

Tuna Casserole

(This recipe seems to have skipped a generation and although we all remember eating it as kids, none of us have the recipe. So here it is.)

1 can of tuna
1 can of cream of mushroom soup
1 small can of chow mein noodles
1 cup of milk
3 tsp. minced dried onions
1 can of mushrooms (drained)
½ box frozen peas (thawed)
crushed potato chips (for topping)

Mix all together in a $13 \times 9 \times 2''$ baking pan and cover with crushed potato chips (now it really feels like the good ol' days), sprinkle with paprika, and bake uncovered for 1 hour at 350 degrees. Serves 6 to 8.

Cereal for Dinner

Open box and pour. Add milk and fruit to taste.

CEREAL FOR DINNER

Adjusting Your Standards
So You Can Heal

⚬ ⚬ ⚬ ⚬ ⚬ ⚬ ⚬ ⚬ ⚬ ⚬ ⚬ ⚬ ⚬ ⚬ ⚬ ⚬ ⚬ ⚬

When one of the breadwinners in a family is "downsized" and is looking for a new job, the rest of the family has to adjust. Everyone has to pitch in. To bridge the gap financially between what they need and what they have, they can spend less, earn more, or a little of both.

It's a similar phenomenon when mommy gets sick. Whether or not mom earns a paycheck, she brings vast resources to the family through her role as head of the family's child-raising, house-cleaning, grocery-shopping and homework-assisting departments, among others. (This varies from family to family but is still a fairly accurate description of most families today.)

So when mommy gets sick—and can't perform at her usual 120 percent level—a gap emerges between what needs to be done and what's possible.

Asking for help, casseroles, car pools, and coverage on a project at work are some great ways to narrow the divide. But there is another tool moms have at their disposal that can be equally effective and even more beneficial in the long run—learning how to adjust (dare I say, lower?) their standards so they can focus on getting well.

This can mean letting your kids watch more TV, letting the dishes pile up in the sink, letting the kids pour their dinner out of a cardboard box. You get the picture. And the good news is that there are ample opportunities to try this out. Think about it: for every set-in-stone rule we have about how we run our household or run our lives, there are equally compelling alternatives that suggest an entirely different approach. As we tinker with our "have-to's" and examine our "shoulds," we'll find a wide array of choices and opportunities to rest.

Here's an example.

Paula had always had very strict ideas about the dangers of watching too much television. Alexandra was only a preschooler when Paula got sick, which meant, among other things, she only went to school in the morning and there were another ten or so hours a day that she was home and needed to be entertained. Early on, Paula had decided that TV would be limited. Alexandra could watch an hour of PBS in the morning before school and then watch two or three hours of cartoons on the weekend. Other than that, the TV was off with the exception of the occasional "movie night" when she, mommy, and daddy made popcorn and watched a movie together.

This was all fine and good when Paula was healthy and could take Alexandra to the park after school, could arrange play dates and have other kids over, and could sit for hours on the floor playing Barbies and Legos with her. But all this changed when she got sick. And one day the insanity of trying to maintain those self-imposed strictures while sick became clear.

I was recovering from surgery and Alexandra was bored.
She was complaining that she had nothing to do but I was
trying to stick to my rules about no TV after school and so I

was hobbling around the house looking for a board game that we could play up on my bed. Well, I almost fainted during the search and when I collapsed on the couch it occurred to me, she's not going to turn into an ax murderer if I let her watch a video after twelve o'clock. So I popped one in and crawled back to bed.

Figuring Out What Really Matters and Forgetting the Rest

What we may find when we're sick is that a lot of our rules and standards are fairly arbitrary. Many of them are simply the by-products of how we were raised. Sometimes we do things exactly the way our moms did. Other times, we seek to parent in an entirely different fashion. Sometimes we form our ideas after talking to friends or base them on something we read in a book, magazine, or newspaper article. Other times, we've sought advice from a pediatrician or other expert. But the fact remains, there are probably as many ways to do the things related to mothering as there are mothers doing them—and most of them are just fine. We simply need to let go.

In my house, this kind of thing shows up whenever Justus is going to be in charge of the kids for any length of time. It's especially bad if he's going to be in charge on a schoolday. Since I work from home, I am the primary lunch-box packer, breakfast maker, and clothes washer in our family. If I am going to be out of this role for a few days, I prepare by leaving notes around the house imparting all my "wisdom" about how things should be. One stuck on the fridge tells him that Travis likes his PB&J folded rather than cut. One next to the calendar reminds him that Addie goes over to Rachel's on Fridays to play after school. Another suggests that he try to get the kids to bathe before dinner so they don't have to go to bed with their hair wet. But, as important as all my sticky notes make this stuff sound, who really cares? He can get along just fine without this information and the kids can get along just fine if daddy does things differently. In fact, they might prefer it.

If, however, I'm stuck in a rigid this-is-how-things-must-be mind-set, everyone else in my family will be too. If I'm not more flexible, how will my kids learn to be flexible and be prepared for life's inevitable inability to satisfy all our needs all the time? The PB&J isn't always going to be folded; the Spiderman T-shirt isn't always going to be clean, and you're not always going to win the election or get the promotion even if you are the most deserving candidate.

Cathy recalls that the biggest adjustment she had to make was letting other parents' rules apply when her daughter was under their care.

> *When my daughter was with other families, their rules were in place. Many of those moms spoke with me first, knowing that I am pretty strict on some things, but I asked them to keep their own routines in place and not worry about my standards.*

Mary Ellen, mother of five grown kids, two of whom still live at home, has been battling cancer for more than a decade. She says it all depends on how she's feeling, but if she had her druthers, she'd never deviate from her high standards.

> *On a good day, if I'm feeling pretty strong, I still try to get dinner on the table so we can all eat together. But on a bad day, everyone has to fend for themselves.*

Darcy, who's got diabetes, two kids, and a full-time job, says it's easy to lower your standards, but the tough part is not feeling guilty about it.

I can let things go for a while, like the house, but after a while I feel bad that it isn't all cleaned up. As for dinners, that's probably where I've made the biggest adjustment. I don't worry anymore that we all try to sit down to a big, home-cooked meal. As long as we eat something relatively healthy at about the same time, I'm pretty happy with that. The reality is that many days I only have enough time and energy to order a pizza or pick up Chinese.

Whether it's not wanting to ask for help or not wanting to lower our standards, women hold tightly onto the reins of "power" in the domestic sphere. We seem to think that by refusing to delegate and demanding that things are done exactly as we specify, we can prove how much we love our families when, in fact, how we can really show that is by taking care of ourselves. We take pride in knowing our children's idiosyncrasies and meeting their needs—but an equally powerful gift is teaching them to accept different approaches and accommodate different outcomes.

And the best way to teach this is to accept that everything isn't always perfect. All of us are truly creatures of habit and we get used to things being a certain way—but it's not always possible. Lowering your standards, changing the routine, shifting your family's expectations when you are sick is a great way to teach your kids how to go with the flow, remind your husband that change is good—and give yourself a break!

Fast Food?
Permission Granted

It has been said that busy moms keep the fast-food industry solvent. Even when we're feeling in top form, life is often too hectic for us to get a well-balanced meal on the table every night—or even four nights out of seven. Sometimes, when the milk is spoiled and we lack the energy needed to rinse out the bowls, even cereal for dinner sounds like too much work. When we get sick, not only do we rely on doorstep dinners and easy-to-serve meals from the pantry, sometimes we have to turn to the Colonel, the pizza guy, and Ronald himself.

To remove any remorse you may be feeling about how many drive-thru meals your kids have had since you got sick, remember again that it is first and foremost *your* health we are worrying about here, not theirs. They will be fine. And like Paula who bent her No TV rule when she realized that her daughter was not going to end up a convict if she watched a bit more television while mommy recuperated from surgery, you can rest assured that you are not condemning your kids to a life of sloth and girth if they eat from restaurants with silly mascots a bit more often when you are sick. (One suggestion during times when fast food is a bigger part of your kids' weekly menu: get them milk instead of soda for their beverage—their bones get the calcium, and they still get the plastic toy.)

Sometimes You Should
Maintain Your Standards
and Keep Your Promises

Once you learn to lower your standards, and everything you do is not done "just because" you've always done it that way or because "that's what moms do," you become better at discerning what things really *do* matter, and what commitments you want to keep even though it might be taxing for you. When we start understanding the difference between options and obligations, the tasks we do take on can bring us great joy—sometimes when we need it most.

Nancy remembered one such occasion.

A week after I got home from the hospital was my daughter's ninth birthday. She was very worried that we would have to cancel the Japanese-themed sleepover party that we had been planning for months. I probably worked a little too hard to get ready so it could go on as planned but it made her feel safer to see me coming through with this promised thing. I was worn out afterwards, but I would do it the same way again if I had to do it over because it brought us both such joy.

WHITE COATS AND WHITE KNUCKLES

Some Thoughts About Dealing with Doctors

◉ ◉ ◉ ◉ ◉ ◉ ◉ ◉ ◉ ◉ ◉ ◉ ◉ ◉ ◉ ◉ ◉

They say only two things are certain—death and taxes. But for a sick mom, I'd add two others—kids and doctors. No matter what else you can delegate, postpone, or ignore, kids and doctors are an omnipresent part of a sick mom's world. And while the presence of our kids can be draining at times, they also provide the love and joy we need to fuel our fight and keep our perspective.

The constant presence of doctors, on the other hand, is not always comforting.

In front of them we are naked, vulnerable, and scared. Because of them our nerves are frayed and our bodies are scarred. Sure, they're trying to save our lives or ease our pain, but that doesn't make it any easier to give control of your body and your day-to-day schedule over to a bunch of people with stethoscopes and lab coats.

Both because we're dealing with the unknown (unless you too went to medical school) and because it interrupts all our normal routines and activities, dealing with doctors can be both daunting and infuriating.

The whole drama of dealing with doctors is one of the most important parts of our illness and recovery. It's also one of the most tangible ways we lose control.

Just like when you take your car to the mechanic and he tells you that your car isn't safe to drive and you need a new transmission. What are you going to say? "No, it doesn't? I'll take care of it?"

Any sense of powerlessness we feel when dealing with doctors can be lessened, I think, by doing some research, taking some of the control back by knowing more about what's going on. When it comes to your car, it's probably not worth the trouble. But when it comes to your *health*, I'd suggest you have no choice.

Stephanie suffers from fibromyalgia, has had cancer twice, and carries with her multipage lists both of the medications she must take daily and the dozens of conditions that she's had to manage for the last twenty years. She is a doctor pro. She says she first learned how to talk to doctors watching her dad at an appointment during the early stages of her cervical cancer.

He asked all kinds of questions and didn't stop until he was satisfied. He probably taught me how to deal with doctors. And thank God he did, because he got me in the habit of asking questions and taking nothing at face value, and that ended up saving my life. After my first cancer surgery, we moved across the country and when I was going to a new doctor I had asked for all my lab reports and files and even I could see from reading them that they hadn't gotten all the cancer out. And no one had even taken the time to read them! So I insisted on getting someone to look at this immediately and when they did they found it had spread like wildfire and then I had to have a total hysterectomy. If I hadn't taken charge, I wouldn't be here today.
—Stephanie

While Stephanie's example may be an extreme one, most of us could use some help in this arena. Here are a few suggestions from the moms I met about how to get what you need from the medical community.

Getting What You Need from Doctors

- ◎ Do as much **research** as possible. Use the library, Internet, bookstore, connect with a support group associated with your condition, talk to friends, etc. If you're not up to the task, this is a great job to delegate to someone who wants to help out. *Note:* information gleaned from the Web is, by definition, general, and not all of it is good. Put it into context and assess its quality by taking it with you to your appointment and discussing it with your doctor. Also, check multiple sources.

- ◎ Draft a list of **questions** and take it with you to your next appointment. If other questions come up before your next visit, jot them down and ask the office manager if you can fax the list over. Tell the doctor or nurse that you might be doing this and would appreciate their help getting you the info you need.

- ◎ Don't be afraid to **probe your doctor's résumé** a bit, especially asking about his or her experience dealing with your exact condition.

- ◎ If you need to make a decision about taking a certain course of action (medicines, surgery, etc.) ask the doctor if you may **speak to another patient** about their decision and its outcomes.

- ◎ If you don't like your doctor, **find a new one**.

⊚ Remember that your doctor got into this line of work because she **wants to help people**. You're her partner and her customer, not her victim.

Now that I am past the worst of my health crisis this list, although long, seems fairly straightforward. But when you're in the middle of it, I know that thinking about this stuff can be overwhelming. It's enough just to schedule and show up at your appointments, much less do all this behind-the-scenes work. But these suggestions can improve both how you're cared for and how you feel about that care.

During the six weeks between my collapse and my surgery, I saw an internist, two neurologists, and two cardiologists. I had a battery of tests including an echocardiogram, treadmill, EEG, EKG, MRI, blood work, and the tilt-table test, and I didn't do a lick of research.

My mom went with me to many of the tests, my husband to the final one. But I didn't research a single thing. I didn't buy a single book or request any information from the American Heart Association. I didn't ask any probing questions.

My worst offense was that even when I did take the time to write down some of my questions before seeing the doctor, I left each appointment with my carefully scribed list still folded neatly and rattling around the bottom of my purse.

We talked about most of this stuff anyway, I'd tell myself as I spied the list while rummaging for my keys by the elevator on my way out.

He seemed to be in a hurry, I'd insist.

She had so many other patients to see, I'd rationalize.

Equally powerful was the shut-down I would experience after I'd worked up the courage to ask one of my questions and received a response. Even if I was still confused, I did not push for any more information—and it's not every doctor who will inquire,

"Do you have any more questions? Is that clear? Does that make sense?" Or, "Is there anything else you would like to know?"

I think the doctor-patient relationship can be particularly challenging for women as the practice of medicine was for years a male domain and women of all but the most recent generations were taught to be pleasant and compliant when dealing with figures of authority such as doctors. Sue, Marty, Paula, and many others said they could relate to the feeling of wanting the doctor to like them and to be seen as a "good patient."

> *I left all the hard stuff to my husband. I didn't want to be difficult. I knew the doctor was doing the best he could for me and I didn't even want to bother him with questions. I did want to be a "good girl." — Paula*

My worst "good girl" moment came when Dr. Jackson walked into the tilt-table room the morning I met him—and the morning he would save my life. Still wanting to believe that there was nothing wrong with me, I considered his presence there a misallocation of talent and resources and a slight to someone who might really need his help.

Certainly there are a lot of people in this hospital that need his expertise much more than I do, I thought, as I lay strapped to the table. *There's lots of old people and sick people here who he could be helping.*

I may not have been old, but I certainly was sick. And moments later Dr. Jackson would use his years of training and well-honed grace under pressure to restart my stopped heart.

Research

Once you go through a serious bout with your health, you become something of an "expert" in several areas where you may have known little before. You learn more than you'd ever want to know about insurance, co-pays, and deductibles, but on the positive side, you come out of it with a better understanding of how your body works and you realize that "medical education" is not just for doctors, but for patients as well.

Thanks in large part to the Internet, patients today are not solely reliant on doctors and other professionals to give them information about their condition but can gather information, pose questions, and seek to further their understanding of what's happening to them on their own. With my condition alone, a simple search begun by my typing "pacemaker" into my AOL search engine nets 11,000 pages or articles and links. Typing in "multiple sclerosis" generates 24,600 pages of results, and even a more obscure condition such as "interstitial cystitis" (a painful bladder disease that strikes mostly women) yields 1,241 pages of relevant sites.

If you don't know where to start, try WebMD and the Mayo Clinic and Johns Hopkins University Medical sites (www.web md.com, www.mayoclinic.com, and www.hopkinsmedicine.org). You can also type just about any disease or condition into a search engine such as www.yahoo.com or www.google.com and come up with reams of information. And if you don't have Internet access (or simply find this whole exercise overwhelming), this is a great thing to ask a friend or relative to do when they tell you (as they will) "If there's anything I can do, don't hesitate to ask." Also, don't overlook the health section at your local library or favorite bookstore. Most also have a section dedicated to women's health.

(Please note that with everything you gather independently, recognize that you should not try to decipher or dissect it entirely on your own. You will need to share it with your doctor and other health-care providers to put it into context. This not only helps you distinguish good information from bad but saves you from the needless worry that will arise if you try to treat and diagnose yourself without proper training.)

You could also ask your partner, sibling, or neighbor to help you go through all the information once it's been gathered. It's too much to do alone and you're going to get tired and depressed doing it, so take it slow and do it with a buddy. One friend likened her experience researching her condition to being in a "war room."

"My husband and I would be at it all night, from the time the kids went to bed until we collapsed from exhaustion. It was intense," she said. "And I never could have done it alone. It was too emotional, too draining, too important."

Questions

Now that you've done your research, it's time to make some lists. Maybe start with a two-columned sheet. On the left side, put "What I Know" and on the other list "What I Still Want to Know." Had I drafted one, my list might have looked like this:

What I Know:	*What I Still Want to Know:*
Sometimes my heart stops beating.	*Why?*
A pacemaker could take care of this.	*Is there any other course of action?*
Surgery is always risky.	*What are the specific dangers associated with this surgery?*
A pacemaker is like a fancy battery	*How does it work? How long does it last? What happens when it runs out?*

A list like this might not fit your style, but one reason I think it works is that it tests what you *think* you know as well as your outstanding questions. The format is not important; the act of writing down your questions is.

Now that you've got your list, put it into action.

- Share it with your "research buddy" to make sure you haven't forgotten anything.

- If you have friends who are doctors, even if they don't specialize in your condition, call them (or have your "buddy" do so) and read them the list and jot down what they have to say. If these conversations lead to more questions, add them to your list.

- If you can prioritize the list, do so and put the most pressing questions at the top.

- Try to get the list as complete as possible because when you show up at your next appointment it's "showtime" and the list is your costar.

The best way to assure that you don't chicken out and skip certain questions—or relegate the entire list to the detritus heap at the bottom of your purse—is to take someone with you to the appointment. And I don't mean just to drive you there and keep you company in the waiting room (although this is nice). I mean someone you know well enough to take with you into the exam room and someone committed enough to act as your advocate in the presence of the doctor. This person also needs to be bold, not afraid of keeping the doctor from her other patients or her golf game if all the questions haven't been answered. I think moms, husbands/partners, siblings, and best friends are good choices. Give him or her a copy of the list and ask them to record the answers so you can focus on listening to the doctor.

Another way to ensure that you use your list is to have a copy for the doctor. Then he or she can see exactly what your questions are and you won't lose your nerve halfway down the list.

It's interesting to observe how your doctor responds to your questions and reacts to your printouts and other research. A doctor who doesn't take your questions seriously or dismisses your attempts to educate yourself on your condition might not be a good fit for you.

Finally, ask the doctor before you leave what's the best way to follow up if you have additional questions before your next appointment. Suggest that you could fax or e-mail additional questions, and ask what he or she would prefer. Ask to be introduced to the head nurse or office manager and tell her that the doctor has suggested the best way to get in touch with him between appointments, and thank her for her help in making sure he gets your messages, e-mails or faxes. By letting them know ahead of time that the doctor is expecting to hear from you, and thanking them for helping make this happen, you ensure less hassle when you call in between appointments. This last part takes a lot of nerve (especially for us "good girls") but it gives you a leg up when you're not in the office but still need the doctor's attention.

Probe Your Doctor's Résumé

When a scary or surprising health-care issue comes up, most people start calling around to get references for a good doctor. If you need a specialist, your internist or primary care doctor will probably recommend one. Depending on your health insurance, you might also have to follow certain strictures when deciding which doctor to see. The American Medical Association also suggests helpful guidelines for finding a good doctor on its Web site (*www.ama-assn.org*) and includes directories with which you can locate doctors based on geography, specialty, or several other factors.

Several moms pointed out to me that their real interest was knowing whether and how their healthcare provider had dealt with their exact conditions and what success she'd had in treating patients with similar profiles. What, they asked, were the different courses of action prescribed in each case and what were the outcomes? The boldest (and smartest?) went a step further and asked if they could meet any of those patients. And that brings me to the next point.

Speak to Another Patient

When my friend Jennie was trying to decide about breast reconstruction after her mastectomy, she asked the surgeon if any of his patients would let her see his handiwork. This meant, of course, finding someone who wouldn't mind taking off her shirt in front of a complete stranger and let her breast be examined. The answer was yes and one woman's generous and intimate sharing encouraged Jennie to go ahead with the surgery.

I didn't have time to talk to any pacemaker patients before undergoing my own surgery (my situation was so critical that they wouldn't even let me leave the hospital until I'd gotten the pacemaker). But I've had the pleasure of being on the receiving end of a few referrals. Twice my cardiologist has sent patients to me to talk about my experience in the hopes of helping them understand their situation and options better. Both were young, otherwise healthy women and it was a gratifying experience for me both times. In one case, the woman brought her mother along so she could meet me and "see" my pacemaker (at least the bump on my chest).

If you can speak on the phone or meet another person who's gone through what you're going through, it makes the whole thing less scary. Among other things, you learn that people can survive the ordeal and it becomes just another part of their life journey.

If You Don't Like Your Doctor, Get a New One

Most of us won't return to a restaurant where the food was lousy or go back to a store where the service was bad, but when it comes to doctors we often feel stuck and feel that we can't make a change. Sometimes it has to do with fatigue and "just wanting to get it over with," but other times it's because we feel like victims more than consumers.

While you may be constrained by your health insurance and other financial matters, you don't have to go to a doctor you don't like. Some women are better at this that others.

✦ *Mothers' Wisdom* ✦

If I don't like a doctor, I just fire him. I don't worry about their feelings. I worry about getting what I need.
—Jacqueline

Between my cancer and my fibromyalgia and everything else that has happened to me, my whole life is doctors. I can't and won't put up with bad service or bad care. My days are just too long for that.—Stephanie

I was horrified with the way I acted around doctors after my accident. I let my husband handle all that and I pretty much just went along with what he and my doctors decided to do. And that's not like me at all. When my dad was sick not long after that, I had to be his caretaker and I was a real bulldog, but for some reason I couldn't do that for myself.—Sue

Doctors Want to Help

I think our relationship with doctors is tricky because so many of us know so little about the inner workings of our bodies. The dynamic can be uncomfortably similar to the feeling we get when taking the car into the shop. The mechanic says we need new brakes, a new water pump, or to have the transmission overhauled, and what are we going to say but "Okay." We wonder the whole time if we're being ripped off or getting the whole story, but we sigh and sign on the dotted line.

But there's an important distinction here. Most doctors really do care and, given the not-so-rosy economic realities of the health-care business today, one can assume that most of those still practicing are doing so for the reason they initially decided to apply to medical school—they're fascinated with the inner workings of the human body and they want to help people live longer, healthier lives.

With only two exceptions, all the doctors I met during my ordeal were intelligent, focused, and had that hard-to-define-but-hard-to-do-without quality called good bedside manner. I am particularly enamored with my internist and cardiologist and when they keep me waiting I try to picture them speaking to patients behind the closed doors that line the hallway and giving each of them the undivided attention I have come to expect when it's my turn.

◉   ◉   ◉

Stephanie, our "doctor pro," has a few tricks up her sleeve that help her get the attention she needs from the many doctors who care for her. She says to treat them as you would personal friends or business associates.

She writes them thank-you notes when she's happy with the care she gets and gives them Christmas presents. She says you always have to do something "to help them remember you." One time she delivered a case of flashy, colored Band-Aids to a doctor who had only the tan "boring" ones. Another time she and a doctor had somehow gotten on the subject of candy, and the next day she sent him a box of his favorites (Fireballs) in the mail. "If they remember me, it will only help the next time I call and need an appointment, need to talk to them at midnight, or need help in a hurry."

She also "fires" doctors who don't meet her standards, and lets them know why. "If I don't like how their staff treated me or kept me waiting, they should know that." She "comparison shops" to find a pharmacy she likes and gets to know the pharmacist on a first-name basis. "The one I have now even gave me his home phone number.

"Look, I'm always at the doctor. I pick and choose which grocery store I go to, why wouldn't I do the same with my health care?"

SCARY STUFF

Waiting for Test Results and Preparing to Go to the Hospital

◦ ◦ ◦ ◦ ◦ ◦ ◦ ◦ ◦ ◦ ◦ ◦ ◦ ◦ ◦ ◦ ◦ ◦

If dealing with doctors is one of the harder parts of being a sick mom, I think it's because we know so little about our bodies and they know so much. We may also see during this crisis that there is even a limit to what they know, and so much of medicine is trial and error, testing and waiting. And as time passes, the fear of *not* knowing is replaced by another fear—that of the knowing—and the inevitable trip to the hospital or clinic for the beginning of "treatment." All scary.

Tests

For a patient, there may be nothing scarier than waiting for test results. Remember waiting to hear from your OB-GYN about the results of your amnio when you were pregnant? Not being able to concentrate on anything else while waiting to hear if the baby you were carrying was free of any major disabilities? Remember having those two weeks drag on as if they were two months and time standing still when the call finally came?

In a world where most things happen at light-speed, time slows to a snail's pace when waiting for the doctor to call. And while this is hard for everyone, it's particularly taxing for moms as we wait for news in the swirling midst of family life with us at the center. While we're consumed with the fear and uncertainty of not knowing what's next for us, we go on making sandwiches, peeling carrots, and sticking little love notes in our kids' lunch bags each morning.

❖ Mothers' Wisdom ❖

When the phone rang with my test results, my daughter's tutor was standing right there with me in the kitchen waiting to be paid. That was weird. She's not the person I would have chosen to be with when I got the news. Certainly that's not how I would have planned it. But you don't get to plan any of this.—Jacqueline

The day I was waiting for the results of my biopsy our neighbor called to see if her daughter could come over to play. I remember thinking, *It's not a great day for a play date because I'm waiting to find out if I have cancer*. But she did come over, and wouldn't you know it, that's when the call came in.—Jennie

I spent the morning we were going to get the lab results back praying, pleading, and begging God to spare my life for the sake of my children. When we got the results I truly felt terror for the first time and thought I was going to pass out. Thank God I could just sit there and have a total meltdown while [my husband] took over.—Jennifer

I had to wait for at least five calls like this in the weeks between my collapse on the bathroom floor and my eventual surgery. First they called to say my heart was fine (and only different tests would later find this not to be true). Then they called to say I didn't have a brain tumor. Next they called to say my bloodwork "revealed nothing of concern."

But then came a call of a different type. The type that starts out with "I'm sorry, but . . ." It was my internist who broke the news to me that I might have epilepsy. I was sitting at the dining room table. I'd worked a half day on a Friday and was home early before the nanny got back from the park with the kids. I'd thought I would get a start on dinner. Instead, I got the call and just sat there in shock. That phone call was my first experience with having my worst fears realized. All the other tests had come back negative. This was a whole new ball game. My internist suggested I get another opinion, but in the meantime, I had to stop driving because epileptics aren't allowed behind the wheel.

A few weeks, and many bus and carpool rides later, the neurologist himself called to say that upon further review he didn't think epilepsy was the cause of my fainting spells. I was relieved, of course, but scared and angry, too. I was thrilled to learn I did not have epilepsy but knew we'd returned to square one and that I'd soon be back on the testing-and-waiting-for-results merry-go-round.

Luckily, we hit the jackpot with the next test and at least this part of my saga was over.

A Few Tips about Waiting for Tests

◉ Spare your kids the drama surrounding the tests. You don't have to tell them you can't see straight because you're so panicked and that you can't go outside and shoot baskets because you can't let the phone out of your sight. Instead, just tell them you're having a bad day so at least they'll understand why you're snapping at every little thing and jumping every time the phone rings.

⊚ Go shopping, or to the gym or out to lunch with a friend. It's good to be distracted. You may miss the phone call but it's sometimes better to have to call back than to have to wait nine hours at home.

⊚ Find something to do with your hands if you have to wait at home for a call. Bake, knit, paint. It helps.

⊚ Understand the way your doctor works. Does she usually make phone calls in between patients? During lunch hour? At the end of the day? The nurses should be able to tell you so you know what to expect.

⊚ Make a list of what you will do if the news is bad. Be specific—who you will call, what you will cancel, what the next steps will be. It helps to have a plan. If the news is good and you get to tear up the list, you won't mind the "wasted time."

⊚ Remember, with test results "positive is negative and negative is positive." (This is the one time when "negative" is what you're hoping for.)

Hospitals

Much can be said about hospitals, but for me they conjure up one single overriding sensation—that of being cold. If you think your doctor's exam rooms with those silly little paper "gowns" are cold, you're right. But they feel like Florida in June compared to the rooms in a hospital. I'm sure there's some medical reason why hospitals have to be kept as cold as an Igloo cooler (probably to keep germs from flourishing) but it's miserable.

When I went to the hospital to have my two kids, I was prepared for the cold. I had a warm robe and my favorite fuzzy socks packed in the overnight case they'd told us about in Lamaze class. But when I arrived in an ambulance the night I collapsed and when I came in via the tilt-table room, I had no time to prepare. I literally had only the clothes on my back, and even these had been taken from me in exchange for the hospital gowns (only slightly thicker than the doctors' paper ones).

I really can't stand to be cold. So I asked the nurse for a sweat-shirt.

The ER nurse said she'd see what she could do and eventually pulled one from the Goodwill box where they kept donated items for indigent patients. It was rose colored with a duck on it. Six weeks later when I found myself unexpectedly back in the hospital, I had the same request. This time I asked my dad. He and my mom had dropped everything and were headed to L.A. upon hearing the news about the tilt-table test and my scheduled surgery. "Do you need anything?" he asked, probably more out of habit than because he actually thought he could do anything to better my dire situation. But there was.

"I need a sweatshirt," I told him. And two hours later I was pulling his big, gray *Sports Illustrated* sweatshirt over my head, over my gown and over the tubes and wires that seemed to be everywhere. No matter, at least I was warm now.

What's your "sweatshirt?" What will make you feel more comfortable when you have to go to the hospital? It may be a CD player with music you like. It may be an afghan from the couch. It may be photos of the kids and crayon-rendered get-well cards. Whatever it is, figure it out and have someone bring it in. Use your judgment, but you probably don't even have to ask if it's okay. In this case, follow the dictum that it's easier to ask forgive-ness than permission. And wait for the nurse or doctor to ask you to turn down the Fleetwood Mac before you self-censor and dis-allow what you think might help you relax.

Fresh berries, a raggedy old puppet, and yoga pants are some of the things that helped other moms I spoke to transform the hospital experience from unbearable to comforting—even if only for fifteen minutes.

❖ Mothers' Wisdom ❖

My mother, who came to see me every day in the hospital, was worried about the amount of weight I was losing so she brought me a bowl of fresh berries and poured half and half and sugar over it. We sat and ate together. I can still remember how good it tasted. How often do you get to drink a bowl of sugary half and half and not feel guilty?—Andrea

When I went into the hospital for my eight-hour surgery, I planned for two main things in the recovery room: a CD player and "Buckwheat." Buckwheat was the name my kids gave to this little neck pillow that I had gotten when we'd flown to Hong Kong. Buckwheat was for my eyes; the CDs were for my ears. They were my ways of blocking out the senses. I used the bunny to fling over my eyes so that I didn't have to see what people were doing to me. And I used the CD player to blast music so I didn't have to hear.—Jennie

Pants! I was more or less confined to bed for the week (though I won an argument with the staff over being allowed to get up to go to the bathroom) and it felt awful to be "in" bed all the time. I really had to wear the stupid hospital gown because it made it easier for the nurses to switch my IV around as needed, but I asked my husband to bring my yoga pants to wear under it. This way I could sort of make the bed and at least spend the days sitting on it outside of the covers. A small thing, but it made a difference.—Nancy

My five-year old packed her favorite puppet into my hospital bag. The puppet is a ragged old bath mitt that belonged to

her older brothers before her. She named the puppet Sockie, and Sockie up until this time always went to bed with her. She was concerned that I would not have any family to sleep with me at the hospital and so Sockie should be there to keep me company. When I came home, I returned Sockie to her and thanked her for thinking of me and sharing Sockie during my time at the hospital. The first day I went back to work, however, my daughter carefully drew a picture of Sockie on a Post-it note and gave it to me as I headed off to work. She was concerned that since I was going back to work, I would still need someone to keep me company.
—Fern

A Few Tips about Hospital Stays

◎ Sure, you know it's not a hotel, but it's not a prison either. Figure out what you need and then ask for it. If the staff can't provide it, ask someone from home to bring it in.

◎ If you've got a semiprivate room and your roommate is loud, difficult, or keeps the TV on all night, ask her to speak more softly or turn off the TV. You can also inquire about switching rooms. The worst they can say is no.

◎ If you know in advance that you're going, plan a little field trip over there with your kids. Don't show them any of the scary stuff, but just walk around the lobby, maybe visit the nursery and peer at the tiny new babies through the glass, buy a trinket in the gift shop or have some Jell-O and hot chocolate in the cafeteria. This will give them a mental picture of where you're going to be, calm their fears, and provide them with positive associations about the hospital.

◎ Whether and when to have your kids visit you in the hospital is a very personal decision best made by you and your husband/partner (or whoever is helping with the kids in your absence). Take into account not only their ages but their personalities, and how they've responded so far to everything that has happened. This—and your "mother's intuition"—will guide you in making the best decision for all involved. You will know the right thing to do. In addition, if your children got to "tour" the facility ahead of time as mentioned above, the need to visit might not feel as urgent and you can then arrange for this important reunion to occur when you're feeling (and looking) your best.

◦ Make a special calendar for your kids (or have a friend do it) marking off the days you're going to be gone and when you're coming home.

Beyond Flowers: What Your Friends Can Bring You in the Hospital that Will Really Make a Difference (*from Jackie, a mom who's been there and knows*)

◦ scented hand and foot lotion—Why use the hospital's generic lotion on your parched skin if you don't have to? Live it up with fancy, silky, great-smelling salves.

◦ flavored lip gloss—The overconditioned air in the hospital wreaks havoc on your lips as well; spread the word about the brands and flavors you like.

◦ a small vase—The big bouquets start to die quickly and your mom, kids, or a pal can clip the longer-lasting flowers and put them in a smaller vase. It might also be nice to have a small vase closer to your bed so you can enjoy their scent.

◦ familiar comfort food—Ask someone who's visiting often to let people know about any cravings, aversions, or doctor-ordered restrictions affecting your diet, and then order up what you're in the mood for. It's also fun to have candy, cookies, and other snacks around to offer visitors who stop by.

◉ Scotch tape and posterboard—Have someone collect the gift cards that come with the flowers and other presents and tape them to a piece of cardboard or posterboard so you can see them up close, keep them in one place, and look at them and feel loved. (If you're a stickler for thankyou notes, you can give this board to a friend and ask her to go to town.)

◉ writing materials—Ask a few friends to bring in pretty stationery and stamps, doodle pads, blank postcards, and markers. You may feel like writing a note or journaling, and it will give you something fun to do with the kids when they come to visit.

◉ fun stuff to read—We're talking *Cosmo, People, Condé Nast Traveler, Vanity Fair*, and *The Oprah Magazine*. Trashy novels, tabloids, and publications like *Sports Illustrated* and *Newsweek* are also nice to have lying around for you to peruse and others to peek at while they're visiting. You can also have fun sharing these with the nurses. Having something else to talk to people about besides your illness is a relief to everyone, you included.

◉ audio gifts—Make sure you've got a Walkman-type portable radio and CD player so you can tune out the noise of the hospital and create your own environment, be it listening to Harry Potter, relaxation CDs, or National Public Radio. Then let people know you're set up to receive and enjoy gifts of music and other delightful, transporting sounds.

◉ fun slippers and socks

◉ bed accessories—Such as a novelty throw pillow, special pillowcase, or cozy afghan to brighten up the room—and your mood.

◉ talking photo frame—From your kids with their picture and their voice recorded. And tell Dad or Grandma that you'd really prefer "We love you, Mom" to "We miss you" or any other message that might be hard to hear when you're away.

◉ stuff off the refrigerator—This one is for your husband and kids. Ask them to go home and take everything off the refrigerator door (the reminder about soccer sign-ups, the lunch menu in the school cafeteria, last year's holiday photo from your sister and her kids) and tape it onto a poster-board and bring it in. It will remind you of all the "regular" stuff still going on and brings a familiar piece of home into the hospital—and don't worry, the fridge will soon be filled up with a slew of other "critical" documents.

(You may want to have a friend make a copy of this list to circulate to all the well-wishers who don't know what to do—and besides, you can never have too much vanilla hand cream or winter-mint lip gloss.)

PART II

∘ ∘ ∘ ∘ ∘ ∘ ∘ ∘ ∘

HOW YOUR ILLNESS
AFFECTS YOUR KIDS

HONESTY

The Benefits of Talking to Your Kids about Your Illness

◦ ◦ ◦ ◦ ◦ ◦ ◦ ◦ ◦ ◦ ◦ ◦ ◦ ◦ ◦ ◦

All of us dislike having to talk to our kids about difficult things. We avoid it by telling ourselves that we are sparing them pain, which never works, because kids find out everything sooner or later. We may say that they won't understand, which is almost never the case, or we use the excuse that a professional should do the telling. But if you can summon the strength to do it yourself, you might find it one of the most fulfilling experiences of your life, one that creates a new strength and closeness between you and your children, one that you will carry with you for the rest of your lives.

—NEIL RUSSELL,
   Can I Still Kiss You? Answering Your Kids' Questions about Cancer
   (Health Communications, Inc., 2001)

Two days before the third anniversary of my surgery, my seven-year-old broke down inconsolably when she learned that I'd be going to New York on business in the coming week. Like most young kids, she likes to have me around and still sometimes clings to my sleeve when I drop her off at school. But this was different. And I wasn't very sympathetic. At least not at first.

Instead, I was irritated.

This will be my first trip out of town in more than a year, I said to myself. *I never go anywhere; can't she just let me go and be happy for me and excited about spending some time with Dad?*

It probably didn't help that this conversation began at the end of the always-longer-than-expected bedtime routine. Luckily, however, I held my tongue, took a deep breath, and probed about why news of this quick trip (across the country and back in less than forty-eight hours) was making her so upset.

In her sweet I'm-not-that-big-yet voice, with tears rolling down her freckled cheeks, she said, "Whenever you leave it's just like when you went to the hospital. It's always like that when you leave and I'm afraid you might not come back."

I couldn't believe it.

Who would have guessed that after three years the memory would be so vivid and the wounds so easily torn open? Clearly, Addie was still recovering emotionally from our shared experience and, I soon realized, so was I.

One of the reasons we were still in the throes of it three years later was that our recovery got off to such a slow start. My kids saw me collapsed on the floor and taken away in an ambulance. My kids saw me lying in a hospital bed hours before surgery "to get a battery to help Mommy's heart."

And my kids saw me come home from the hospital and pretend nothing had happened. I mistakenly thought that talking about what had happened during or after the fact would only make it worse. It was just the opposite.

My conversations with the moms in this book revealed that when, what, and how much your kids know about your illness will vary greatly depending on your condition. They provided the following advice:

◎ For moms with cancer, there will probably be "the big talk" sometime soon after the doctor first utters the "C word." Then there will need to be ongoing conversations as treatment progresses.

◎ For moms with multiple sclerosis, their kids may not need to know much at first (especially if they're young and mom's symptoms are mild) but as the disease progresses, they will have to be told when mom is grappling with new symptoms and a decreased range of motion. They'll also come to know the difference between her "good days" and "bad days" because she'll talk to them about both.

◎ For moms with diabetes, conversations may focus on nutrition, ups and downs in blood sugar and energy level—and how needles and medicine are a part of life.

◎ For a mom with an autoimmune disease such as lupus or fibromyalgia (or even periodic but severe migraines), kids will learn to understand mommy might be in a lot of pain even if she "looks just fine."

Whatever the circumstances, whatever the condition, experts agree that you must not hide your illness from them. You may say a lot, you may say a little, but you should say something. And then be prepared for their questions, fear, and anxiety, even while dealing with your own.

"Kids are exquisitely sensitive to the emotions of adults. Their survival actually depends on their ability to perceive non-verbal cues and to read the social and emotional states of their caregivers. For this reason, children can be more frightened by the fear and anger of their caregivers than they are by what's actually happening.
—Dr. Peter Levine, Ph.D., *It Won't Hurt Forever: Guiding Your Child Through Trauma*

Kids' Sixth Sense

The consensus from counselors, teachers, early childhood experts—and the moms I've met who've been there—is that it's important to get things out into the open with your children for several reasons:

1) They're going to know something's going on.
2) They will be less afraid if they don't have to try and eavesdrop on whispered phone conversations or decipher the muffled words of people talking behind closed doors.
3) Children think in black and white, and unless you put the matter into context, they will think the worst.
4) Your kids will need some outlet for their fear and anger, and without a forum to talk about it at home they will either internalize it or start acting out at school and elsewhere.
5) Just like the better-sooner-than-later talks about drugs, alcohol, and the birds and the bees that are a required part of parenting, it is better to be proactive in providing information about mommy's condition than waiting for your kids to try to figure it out on their own.

Kids have this thing where they just know if something is wrong, even if their mom and dad aren't saying anything. I think kids have a right to know because they don't want to feel alone and they want to help. But they can't help if no one tells them what's going on.
—Taylor, *age ten, whose mom has diabetes*

Emotional Hide-and-Seek

One of the hardest things about being a sick mom is that you're always being watched. Even when your kids are pretending they don't hear you asking them to turn off the TV, wash their hands, and come to dinner, they usually have a pretty good idea where you are, what you're doing, and how you're feeling. And while they may act as if your emotional state is none of their concern, this is just a ruse. I've seen hundreds of times how my bad mood can infect the whole family and how my happiness can lift everyone else's spirits. So when it comes to something as serious as your health, something that's going to affect your mood whether you like it or not, you won't be able to pretend everything's fine when in fact you're scared to death.

During the month-long limbo between my trip to the ER and my diagnosis and surgery, I don't remember a single conversation with them explaining what was going on or addressing what I know was a pervading sadness and fear in the house that I was trying to mask with activity and an ardent things-are-just-fine performance.

"Kids know what's going on. They're going to feel the parent's stress, anxiety, and fear," says Lynette Wilhardt, LCSW, clinical director and program manager of Kids Konnected, a national support group for children who have a parent with cancer.

"A parent who's not talking about it is not [acknowledging] the experience, so kids are just at a loss as to what's going on, and that makes it all the more difficult for them to cope."

Thinking I was "sparing them" undue worry about an illness that had not yet been identified, I pretended everything was normal when that was far from true. I can tell myself that the problem was that I had no time to prepare, role-play, or rehearse, that things just happened too quickly, but I think there's another reason.

I was scared. And if I admitted to them that I was sick, I would have to admit it to myself.

Six months after my surgery, six months after I almost died, you wouldn't have known anything had ever happened. I'd been back at work for months, taking on more and bigger assignments. Justus and I were planning a trip to Cabo San Lucas to celebrate our tenth wedding anniversary, our nanny had just quit, and the kids were acclimating to their new one. Our lives had returned to the familiar swirl of activity. There was just one problem, just one sign that I was not as okay as I made out to be. I was yelling at everyone—especially the dog and the kids. One night after a particularly taxing pajamas-brush-your-teeth-read-the-story-and-please-get-to-bed episode, Justus and I sat collapsed on the couch. I wondered out loud why the kids had been so difficult of late and "why was everything so hard," and he looked right into my tear-filled eyes, and said, "I think you have a virus on your spirit." I don't remember what I said next. I hope I was not defensive. But like Jenny's call to 911, this was one of those before-and-after moments. And thus began my long search to come to terms with what had happened and how it might be affecting me, the kids, my marriage, my life.

I wanted to believe that refusing to talk about my illness and fear would make it go away. Of course I knew better, but I couldn't act on that knowledge. I was paralyzed. It was like the elephant standing in the corner of the room that no one has acknowledged. Finally, someone had to say something. And when at last we did admit that we'd been through something traumatic, we could begin to heal. Indeed, our emotions needed tending long after my physical condition had been stabilized. I just wish someone had pointed this out to me, but I would have to find out for myself, and, luckily, it wasn't too late.

A Gift from Beyond

Having witnessed her own mother's battle with cancer while in her late teens, Jennifer had painful but powerful experience to draw upon when she was diagnosed with breast cancer and contemplated how to talk with her young kids about illness and death. The pain of the past morphed into a plan for the present and allowed a gift to pass from Jennifer's mom to the grandkids she never knew by way of a mother/daughter who had learned a most powerful lesson.

> *When my mother was diagnosed with multiple myeloma, a kind of blood cancer, I was seventeen years old and beginning my senior year of high school. I was horrified at the diagnosis but really believed that she would get better. Maybe because of that, I was not very sympathetic. I did not understand why she was so sick with her chemotherapy and did not cut her a lot of slack. I was impatient and angry and refused to accept the fact that she was not able to be the mother or person that I needed and that I had become used to. Remember, I was seventeen and pretty much felt the world revolved around me.*
>
> *When she showed initial response to the chemo, I was elated and was sure that it was a sign she was cured—and that I would have "my old mom" back. And in a way I did. The cancer was in remission and life returned to normal.*
>
> *Then she had a recurrence. By this time, I had grown up a bit and was more in touch and less angry. However, I still was not the support to her that I could have been in terms of calling or visiting. I was away at college and was busy with my studies, part-time work, and extracurricular activities. We spoke about once a week on the phone and I would visit*

about once a month when I had the chance. Although we both knew she was dying, we never spoke of it, we never cried together, not even once.

I regret this with all my heart because I missed out on a part of my mother I can never have back. Of course, she set the tone of things we were able to talk about, being the mother and being the one who was ill. She did not bring it up and I followed her lead. I wanted to share my heart and soul with her, wanted to talk about it, but was so afraid that voicing my deepest, darkest fear would somehow make it so.

I wish we'd both had more courage and talked about what was happening. I wish she had initiated these talks. She probably felt the same as I did. It was just too much of a hurdle for us to get over.

She always did her best to be positive, cheerful, and outwardly focused when we were together, even to a fault. She never wanted to speak of her coming death and worsening condition. She always wanted to hear of my classes, fellas I was dating, etc. I wish she had let us talk more about her illness instead of changing the subject.

When we did speak of her death toward the end, including the day she died, it was terse and matter-of-fact. There was little emotion, although it was tearing me up inside. I wish things could have been different.

I cannot speak for every child, but if I could go back and give my mother some advice on how to handle things with her nearly grown children, it would be to initiate and show emotion. It is okay. Not doing so will deprive your family of a part of you that will not be there after you are gone. It will help them heal faster, having shared something so vulnerable, fragile, and even beautiful together.

Nothing can ever replace the moments I lost with my mother, but perhaps my experience will help another family to deal with this unspeakable tragedy together. Although my

girls are young, it has already helped me and given me
strength and courage to talk to them about my cancer, even
about the scary stuff.
—Jennifer

Not talking to my kids is my single biggest regret about my health crisis and recovery. I'll do it differently next time (for there's bound to be another health "bump" down the road for one or more of us) and I encourage *you* to consider talking to your kids now and save yourself a big blow-up later, or lots of regrets and guilt about how you could have handled your crisis differently.

Moms dealing with chronic, rather than acute, illness, may be tempted not to "bother" their kids with too much information about their condition. If you have diabetes or MS, lupus, or fibromyaligia, you may think that the less said the better because you're probably not in imminent danger and your illness is just "part of life" that everyone is going to have to get used to. Darcy, Grace, and Shelley all recall feeling this way. But, they say, in these cases talking to your kids might be even more important because they will have to come to understand the progressive or lasting nature of your condition and how you may need their help to make sure you are taking care of yourself. With chronic illness, it is not only you who have to adjust but the whole family—and to do so, your kids need to be in the loop.

⊙   ⊙   ⊙   ⊙   ⊙   ⊙   ⊙   ⊙   ⊙   ⊙   ⊙   ⊙   ⊙   ⊙   ⊙   ⊙   ⊙

I know a lot about it, really. She tells us the things we need to
know about diabetes so we can help her. We all work together to
keep Mom healthy.
—Taylor, *age ten, whose mom has diabetes*

⊙   ⊙   ⊙   ⊙   ⊙   ⊙   ⊙   ⊙   ⊙   ⊙   ⊙   ⊙   ⊙   ⊙   ⊙   ⊙   ⊙

For me, although the danger has passed and my treatment now consists primarily of quarterly pacemaker checks to monitor how much juice is in the battery and annual visits to my cardiologist, it's still a part of our day-to-day lives.

Even though I am no longer in crisis, my condition is a member of the family that demands to be acknowledged.

So now I tell them when I am going to the doctor, and give them the report when I return. I don't think they fully understand that I have to get the pacemaker replaced every five to seven years, but as the date approaches, we will prepare together for mommy's next surgery.

Just as their fear was ever-present when I was in denial and not talking to them about my illness, their sense of peace increases every time I let them into and make them a part of my healing, maintenance, and recovery. The same is true for your family.

Many of the symptoms associated with cancer, MS, diabetes, fibromyalgia, and other conditions are not visible to the human eye. How, then, do you describe fatigue to your five-year-old? How do you explain to your teenager that you're in too much pain to get out of bed? Below are a few tips for talking to kids about the things they cannot see in a way they might understand.

1) **Explain that your energy supply is like a bank account.** You have a certain amount to "spend" each day, so it's up to you to decide when and how you're going to use it. Saving the hardest jobs for when you have the most energy, not spending what you have all at once, planning (and saving), for those times when you know you'll need more energy, are just a few ways to manage your "account" wisely.

2) **Try to relate what you're feeling to things they may have experienced.** For example, "Remember when you had that really bad tummy ache and you were throwing up all night? That's how mommy feels all day long. That feeling is called "nausea." Or "Remember how tired you were after you stayed up late to go to watch that movie and then

you had to go to school the next day? That's how mommy feels all the time, even after I take a nap."

3) **Get comfortable with it being uncomfortable.** As mothers, we spend a lot of time meeting our kids' needs and making things easy for them. This is just not always going to be possible when we are sick. They may get mad. They may stomp off or go away moping and shuffling their feet when they think you're being unfair. But you can't spend too much of your precious energy managing their moods. Regardless of what they can see with their eyes and what their perception may be of your illness, only you know how you're feeling and you have to set ground rules that give you the best chance at resting and recovering.

WARNING SIGNS

Knowing When Your Illness
Is Troubling Your Kids

◎ ◎ ◎ ◎ ◎ ◎ ◎ ◎ ◎ ◎ ◎ ◎ ◎ ◎ ◎ ◎ ◎

Addie had just turned four when my crisis hit. She had always been a cheerful, bubbly child with a don't-worry-be-happy demeanor.

After I got sick, this changed.

She became quiet and timid. She often didn't want to go to school and when she was there she was withdrawn and primarily interacted with her brother and one other friend. She was easily brought to tears and often ran to hide under her bed when she was ashamed, afraid, or confused, and it was a real feat to coax her out.

As dramatic as this change was, it took me months to make the connection between these changes and my illness. I never stopped to see it through the eyes of a tiny little girl who saw her mother collapse and be driven away in a speeding ambulance. I never considered how scary it must have been to be told that there was something wrong with her mom's heart, and how being told "mommy's heart needs a battery" probably wasn't a very comforting thought. After all, kids know from an early age that batteries don't last forever.

A few months after my operation, Addie's preschool teacher pulled me aside and told me that Addie seemed to be having a hard time at school and she asked if there might be anything going on at home that would account for this. Even then, I was clueless. I suggested that it might be the fact that our longtime nanny had quit and the kids were adjusting to a new baby-sitter. Sure, this *was* an adjustment for the kids. But the real problem was all her pent-up anxiety and all the unanswered questions she had that related to my illness.

Experts suggest that everything Addie was doing was normal, internalizing fear and anxiety about what was going on around her—especially because no one was talking about it. They point out, of course, that children will react differently depending on their personalities and other factors, but that a reaction of some sort is inevitable. In many cases, the changed behavior will be most evident at school or in other settings where mommy isn't present. At home, the troubled child may be withdrawn. At school he may act out. A child may lose interest in activities that used to thrill her, may be easily distracted at school when normally she is an avid learner, may want to spend time alone in her room, or away from home busying herself with friends and outings. Boys may get angry. Girls may be moody.

All of this is normal. But it can be lessened by providing an open forum for communication—and it can be exacerbated if everyone is afraid to talk.

❖ Mothers' Wisdom ❖

Without being too dramatic, I definitely saw signs of trauma in how my kids reacted to my illness. My daughter missed a lot of school in the weeks following my initial illness and would often visit the school nurse complaining of chest pains and shortness of breath. These were the symptoms I was displaying. We checked with our pediatrician just to make sure nothing was wrong with her and confirmed what we thought all along—that she was using these complaints as a way to work through her fears about what was happening to me.—Nancy

[My son] was sixteen when my diagnosis occurred. He's always been more communicative than most, but he was still a male adolescent and pretty tight-lipped. We took a long-planned trip to Europe after my surgery and before my radiation treatment was set to begin. We were in the basement of the Pantheon where the tombs of lots of famous folks are located and he stopped in front of the tomb of Madame Curie (who some call the mother of radiation) and put his arm around me, and said, 'Thank God for Madame Curie. If not for her, Mom, you wouldn't have a chance.' It was a touching reminder that even though we weren't talking about it, my illness was at the top of his mind.—Marty

My kids' reactions were not subtle at all. They were scared of me when I got home from the hospital and literally ran away from me. Not only was I totally laid up and unable to do anything for myself or for them, I had contracted a grotesque rash on my face while in the hospital and they didn't even want to look at me. They stayed away and only wanted to be with my husband or my mom. It was one of the hardest things about my illness. It took a while before we all figured out how to relate to each other again.—Andrea

My ten-year-old can understand intellectually the course of the disease and often shows great signs of compassion when he sees my struggles. My four-year-old is trying to get a handle on the unpredictability of it. I think sometimes he wants to test my claim that I have this disease that makes me tired, trip easily, weak in the heat, or clumsy, and other times he says he'll be my cane, and helps me climb difficult curbs or other challenges.—Grace

An article by Elsie Hsieh in *Family Matters* (winter 2002), a special issue of *MAMM* (a magazine for breast and reproductive cancer patients), cites several studies and gives some great advice about how kids might react to news that their mom has cancer. I think her counsel is relevant and helpful for all moms, regardless of their condition.

Here are a few summary points:

⊚ Before age six, children can only comprehend the most basic information about your disease and are less likely to have an emotional reaction because they don't really understand about death. They often believe the condition is reversible and their concerns will probably center on how your illness will affect them (e.g., "How come mommy can't play with me right now?")

⊚ From seven to twelve, it is common for children to exhibit strong emotional reactions and separation anxiety, believing somehow that if they stay by your side you will be okay and nothing (not even death) will take you away. They may want to skip school and may be very attentive and clingy. In addition to social withdrawal, children in this group may experience depression, anger, and mood swings.

⊚ Teenagers' overriding concern is fitting in with peers, and anything that makes them feel different can cause them to respond with anger, frustration, or apparent uninterest. Depending on the child, teens will either want to know everything or nothing about mom's illness.

No one knows your kids better than you and no one has instincts like a mom. So if you've got your antennae up and are aware that your kids may be struggling or concerned because of your illness, you won't miss it.

And, like Addie's breakdown when I was headed out of town on business, there doesn't appear to be any "statute of limitations" on these feelings. It was just a few weeks after that talk that another one was started. This time by Travis.

"It sure is good you have that battery, Mom," he offered one night as we were finishing up the night's bedtime story. "Because if your heart doesn't beat, then you die." (I found out later that his kindergarten class had been studying about the heart that day in school.)

Then Addie chimed in.

"Yeah, and kids really need their mommies—even when they're big."

Message received. Loud and clear.

Taking care of me *is* taking care of them.

TOOLS FOR TALKING

The ABCs of Talking to Your Kids and Calming Their Fears

◉ ◉ ◉ ◉ ◉ ◉ ◉ ◉ ◉ ◉ ◉ ◉ ◉ ◉ ◉ ◉

The day my family found out my mom had breast cancer, everything was so messed up. There were a gazillion phone calls, my mom and dad were whispering, and I even heard my mom crying. I wasn't sure what was going on but I knew it wasn't good. I was scared. Nothing got done that day. My mom didn't do the weekly grocery shopping (so I ate cookies for dinner!). My iguana, Sydney, got loose; my dad put the milk in the pantry; and my sister went to sleep in her tutu. My house was never crazy like that before.

—ANTHONY, age eight

We sure needed (family meetings) when my mom started treatment. . . . Meetings help everyone in my family talk to each other: Mom and Dad explain the new rules, like who takes out the garbage or who puts the dishes in the sink. Talking with my family helps me understand what's going on and makes me feel better and a lot less lonely. Now I feel like we're on the same team. You don't have to have special meetings to talk, but if you

*do, you might end up with a snack. We like peanut butter chip
cookies.*

—Miguel, age seven
—*The Hope Tree* by Laura Numeroff and Wendy S. Harpham,
   M.D.

Whether you're trying to muddle through those first
"messed-up" days or baking cookies in anticipation of
your next "family meeting," a little preparation can go a long
way when it comes to helping your kids make sense of your illness. Here are some tips gleaned from my favorite books, experts, and friends:

What to Do
Right Now

- ⊚ **Prepare** to talk to your kids by talking first to your husband or partner about when and how you want to explain
  to your kids about your illness. If possible, plan to have the
  initial talk as a family with everyone present. Keep your
  language simple but honest.

- ⊚ **Be a learner.** If possible, consult books, brochures, and the
  Internet for answers to some of the basic questions your
  kids might ask. Those who've gone before us and professionals who work with kids and families have much to
  teach.

- ⊚ **Prepare your kids for the changes in daily routines** that are
  likely while you're sick, mending, and seeking treatment,
  and tell them that being flexible (like eating a meal brought
  by a neighbor even if it's not their favorite) is going to help
  mommy rest and feel better faster.

- ◉ Think about finding appropriate **ways for them to help**.

- ◉ **Inform their teachers** about what's going on at home.

- ◉ **Let your kids know you're available to talk** and that they can ask for a family meeting anytime they think they need one, and that they should continue to ask questions and talk about how they're feeling as they go about their daily routines.

Preparing for the Talk

After you, who knows your kids best? Is it their dad? Is it a grandparent, aunt or uncle, family friend or special teacher? Figure it out and enlist that person's support as you prepare to talk to your kids. If the person you choose does not live with you (your ex-husband, grandma, or a favorite uncle) it's critical that you bring him or her into the loop. The last thing your kids need is conflicting information or mixed signals during this scary time. It helps if everyone who's close to the kids is in sync. If you and your husband no longer live together, ask him to be there so your kids can see that the family is coming together around mommy's illness and there's plenty of love and support to go around.

In preparing to talk to your kids, you'll have to be willing to go to some of the "dark places" where you may not have gone on your own. That's because kids rarely deal in nuances or niceties, especially when they're scared. They're going to say exactly what's on their mind, ask exactly what pops into their head. Such as, "Do people die from that? Are you going to die?" In fact, studies that have been done about how kids are impacted by a parent's illness suggest that the number-one reason adults do not talk honestly with their kids about what's going on is that they aren't prepared to field questions about death.

By age six, most children understand that everyone dies. If your condition truly is life threatening, you can tell them that "people die from lots of things, but I don't think I am going to die from this. I have a lot of really nice and really smart doctors helping me so that I can get better." Consulting with counselors and others who have "been in your shoes" will help tremendously when looking for answers to these questions.

The following Q & A comes from Neil Russell's book, *Can I Still Kiss You?* and offers a nice example.

Q. Do people die from cancer?

A. Unfortunately, some people do. But others are treated successfully. Those people can then lead normal, happy lives.

Q. Are you going to die?

A. The doctors are going to do everything they can to make me well again, but sometimes things can happen that no one wants or expects.

Q. What will happen to me if you die?

A. It will be a difficult time, but we have a very strong family, all of whom love you very much. If I do die, they will be there to take care of you.

This dad's simple, honest, and loving approach to answering the most profound questions of all serve as a great model from which all of us can craft a message that is both truthful and comforting.

This kind of dialogue sets the tone and makes it clear that the lines of communication are open and that everyone's feelings, fears, and questions are valid and welcome. Having started this way, you can fall back on the model time and time again, both as your illness and recovery progress, and in other times of family crisis (the death of a close relative, divorce, even the loss of a job).

In circumstances where your life is not in danger, you should certainly say that right off the bat. "Mommy is going to be tired and I'm going to have to go to lots of doctors appointments, but you don't have to worry that I am going to die from this. Sometimes it might hurt and sometimes I might cry, but I know I will get better."

❖ *Mothers' Wisdom* ❖

My kids all reacted differently, and in each case it fit their personality. For my son, who is very into math and numbers, he wanted to know facts and percentages. Once we could tell him something like "The doctors said there's a ninety percent chance they got all the cancer out," he was fine. For my daughters, it was more emotional, and to this day, two and a half years later, they are very aware of everything they see that has to do with breast cancer. They clip articles, they pull the lids off the yogurt cartons during Breast Cancer Month, and out of the blue they'll hug me and say, "I'm glad you're better, Mom." It will just come up for them when I'm not even thinking about it. I don't think it's ever far from any of our minds actually.
—Jacqueline

Learning from Others' Experience and Expertise

When it comes to developing materials to help patients talk to their kids about their illness, the cancer community has done the best job and produced the most. This is probably because death looms large in any discussion about the disease. It is a shame, however, that there isn't as much published about the impact of other illnesses on mothers, children, and family dynamics. Here's some of what I've found, and you'll find some other tips and suggestions in the Resources section at the end of the book:

- MSMoms.com for mothers with multiple sclerosis

- *Keep Smyelin,* a quarterly newsletter for kids who have a parent with MS, available from the National MS Society at 1-800-FIGHTMS

- Diabeticmommy.com for moms and their kids dealing with diabetes

- Fibrohugs.com is a site offering support, resources, and opportunities to meet other moms with fibromyalgia

- *The Hope Tree,* a picture book for kids whose moms have cancer, published by Simon & Schuster Books for Young Readers

- KidsKonnected.com is an organization for children who have a parent battling cancer

- Rainbows is a twenty-year-old organization for kids and families struggling with loss, grief, and other 'life-altering crises' (www.Rainbows.org)

Once I started talking about what happened, my kids knew that they could too, and as things were brought out into the open, they were put in context and suddenly everything wasn't as scary. One of my most memorable exchanges with Addie related to my illness came right after Valentine's Day, right after Justus identified the "virus on my spirit." We started out talking about issues of life and death. We ended up talking about Barbie.

"Why does your heart need a battery?" she asked.

"Sometimes when my brain tells my heart to beat, the message doesn't get through." I said. "So this battery is always on and can send the message loud enough so that my heart always hears it. So we don't have to worry that that will ever happen again."

Satisfied with this answer, she turned around, picked up her Glamour Barbie, and said, "Wanna play?"

If we think we can't put ourselves first because our kids won't be able to adjust, if we think we can't tell them what's going on because they will be devastated, if we think we have to sacrifice our needs for theirs—think again. If we've built a foundation of love and then reinforced it by talking with them truthfully and sharing with them honestly, our kids are never more than one conversation away from asking us to take them to the mall, telling us what toy is in the Happy Meal this week, or sharing with us the latest gossip from school.

✔ TRY THIS

Take a shoe box, cut a hole in the lid, and have the kids decorate the outside of the box with glitter, collage, or markers. Have the kids tape or staple an envelope on one side. On the top of the box, write "Talk Box." Buy a pack of colored index cards and put the blank cards in the envelope. Ask the kids to write down feelings, questions, and complaints they have about what's going on and all the changes around the house and tell them you're going to open the box once a week and go through the cards as a family. Little ones can dictate their entries to mom, dad, or an older sibling.

HEAVY LIFTING

Conversations about Death and Dying

⊚ ⊚ ⊚ ⊚ ⊚ ⊚ ⊚ ⊚ ⊚ ⊚ ⊚ ⊚ ⊚ ⊚ ⊚ ⊚ ⊚ ⊚

The Barbie conversation with Addie surprised me because I wouldn't have suspected, not in a million years, that she'd move so quickly from contemplating death to considering what gown her long-legged doll would wear for that day's escapades. It revealed to me that a little information can go a long way with children and that, no matter what the news is, kids would rather hear it straight up than be left to sort through their fears and questions on their own.

Again and again, experts and moms and dads in the trenches have told me that even a talk about death and dying, if prepared for thoughtfully, can be a great relief to kids in a household where mommy is sick.

John, whose wife, Louise (also my dear friend and college roommate), died of a rare form of B-cell lymphoma at age thirty-five, said this was his experience as he and Louise prepared their two children for the inevitability of her death.

> *The thing that surprised me the most was that when we
> finally told [our six-year-old son] that mommy wasn't going
> to get better, that she was going to die, it was almost like he
> was relieved. He was really sad, but I think he knew before
> we did. He was very tuned in to Louise and into what was
> going on and I think it was a great weight off his shoulders
> when we told him because he no longer had to carry the
> burden of all that fear and wondering on his own.*

John's intimate sharing about this most challenging of all family moments provides some valuable insights. In his experience, the prospect of telling the kids proved worse than the reality. His story suggests that facing the issue head-on gives everyone the chance to process their feelings, ask the questions they've been afraid to ask (e.g., "Who's going to take care of me?" and "What if daddy dies too?") and begin together to build a plan for grieving and beyond. John says he thinks Louise lived as long as she did (almost three years—which was two years longer than doctors expected) because "she wanted to help us get ready. She wanted to make sure that I could handle it and that I knew everything I'd need to know to carry on without her."

That sounds just like Louise—and just like every other mom I know—multitasking and taking care of things until the very end. Indeed, accepting news of their own mortality is much easier for most moms than picturing how their husband and little ones will go on without them, and they want to help in any way they can while there is still time. This is neither selfless nor overly self-important. It's simply a conscious recognition of the vast place a mother occupies in the life of her family.

For families with a strong faith tradition, this can be a time of prayer and contemplation of heaven and other concepts of what happens after we die. Every religion has its own answer to this, the biggest mystery of all, and now is a good time to share your beliefs with your children or explore together the many different ways this question has been answered by different cultures in different times. John says, "church and faith" were what got his children through the initial crisis—and what still help them today.

> *They can always fall back on their religion. I was able to tell them from the beginning that they would see their mom again and that she's watching over them until that time. I tell them that we're only here for a short time and that mommy already passed the ultimate test and got to go live with God.*

In the years since my brush with death, the subject comes up more and more. The kids feel free to talk about it, and even know that mommy and daddy have different ideas about what happens after we die, giving them a chance to contemplate our ideas and others to come up with their own understanding. What's most important and comforting to them is that daddy's more traditional Christian concept of heaven in the clouds and my more New Age belief in reincarnation both include a loving higher power and the expectation that we'll all be together again, whether as angels or sea otters, no matter when or how we leave this earth.

Elise NeeDell Babcock, author of *When Life Becomes Precious* and founder of Cancer Counseling, Inc., says,

> *Although you may want to protect your child by not giving her bad news, keeping information from her will cause even more problems. By telling her in age-appropriate ways, you are building trust. You can be honest, upbeat and realistic while telling them how mommy is doing each step of the way. And, most importantly, let children grieve and reassure them of your love. Let them know there will always be someone to care for them.*

Many parents turn to books and other outside resources to help them prepare for this most important of all conversations and to try to simplify, demystify, and lessen the pain around the subject of death for their kids. Parents will find many practical suggestions in Babcock's book. One chapter deals specifically and effectively with sharing the news with your kids, and includes a twenty-one-point list of things to consider as you prepare for the talk (e.g., teach your children to hope for something other than a cure; be comfortable saying "I don't know," and be prepared for anger.) Another book to check out is *How to Help Children Through a Parent's Serious Illness* by Kathleen McCue.

You can find an array of other helpful books in the psychology and self-help section of your local bookstore or library or by typing keywords such as "grief" into the search index on Amazon.com and other Internet booksellers.

You might also want to find books written for a younger audience that you can read with your kids during this difficult time. A few examples include:

- *The Fall of Freddie the Leaf*, by Leo Buscaglia

- *Sad Isn't Bad: A Good-Grief Guidebook for Kids Dealing with Loss*, by Michaelene Mundy

- *What's Heaven?* by Maria Shriver

- *Help Me Say Good-bye: Activities for Helping Kids Cope When a Special Person Dies*, by Janis Silverman

- *Lifetimes: A Beautiful Way to Explain Death to Children*, by Bryan Mellonie

- *Where Does God Live?* written by Rabbi Marc Gellman and Monsignor Thomas Hartman

- *Healing the Hurt, Restoring the Hope*, by Suzy Yehl Marta, founder of Rainbows

It was suggested to me once that books like these be a part of your family library and bedtime reading repertoire even when there is no crisis looming or just past, as it shows kids that suffering and death are nothing more than another part of life. I think this is a lovely idea.

Finally, several families and grief experts suggested things that a sick mom might want to do if and when she learns that her death is imminent. They include:

◉ **Writing an ethical will.** This practice has a long history in the Jewish religion but has gained wider popularity, and a search on the Internet now provides numerous links to books, workshops, and chat groups. A good place to start is *www.ethicalwill.com*. Like it sounds, an ethical will identifies the values that you want to pass on to your children and is not a legal document but a statement of what you believe in and how you believe it can help the loved ones you leave behind. As is the tradition, writers of these wills are encouraged to share them with their families before they die.

◉ **Recording your voice.** Surely there are photographs of you and the kids all around the house (and take more if there are not), but other than your voice on the answering machine, there may be no recordings of your voice. Choose something special to read (one of the kids' favorite books, a poem, a personal message to each child) and get it onto a tape (or CD if you know how to do that). Some families choose to do a video recording as well, although it may be harder to watch than listen to mom after she's gone.

◉ **Writing letters.** These pieces can take many forms. Louise chose to write individual letters to each of her kids commenting on aspects of their emerging personalities that she found most endearing and her hopes and dreams for their future. Other moms choose to write letters to be opened in the future on special occasions such as birthdays, prom night, weddings, and the birth of a child. Others write minibiographies and put down on paper special memories from their own childhood that they'd like to share.

◉ **Creating a mommy box.** Send someone out to buy a fancy box, maybe a lacquered wooden one or one made of porcelain or stone (alternately, you can use a decorated shoe box). Put it in a special place in the house and tell the kids that this is going to be their "mommy box" and that when they have something that is bothering them or that they are worrying about after mommy's gone, they can write it down, and put it in the box and know that she is going to help them take care of it.

◉ **Buying balloons, ribbon, and notecards.** Like the mommy box, this idea speaks to the kids' need to do something physical to make contact with mom after she's died. Let the kids know that they can send a prayer, wish, or problem up to mommy via a helium-filled balloon. This idea came from a six-year-old classmate of Louise's son who was sad that he couldn't give his mommy a handmade card on Mother's Day. It has since become their family's annual tradition to send cards aloft, and leaves the kids beaming from ear to ear.

PARTNERSHIP

What Your Kids Can Do for You

⊚ ⊚ ⊚ ⊚ ⊚ ⊚ ⊚ ⊚ ⊚ ⊚ ⊚ ⊚ ⊚ ⊚ ⊚ ⊚ ⊚

*Y*our kids' main job is to keep being kids even when mommy gets sick—and maybe *especially* when mommy gets sick. Things will be heavy enough around the house without them feeling as though they can no longer laugh, be silly, or make a mess. Especially with older children (teen and preteen girls in particular), you want to guard against their taking on an undue sense of responsibility for running the household, taking care of younger siblings, or meting out chores or discipline. They need to understand that your illness is a problem they did not create and a situation they will not be able to make go away. That said, there are certain things they *can* do that will help you get the rest you need and satisfy their need to feel that they're contributing to your healing.

Your kids can help most by:

◎ being flexible

◎ being patient

◎ being honest

◎ being on the team

Asking Your Kids to be Flexible

If the main thing *you're* going to need to get through this is courage (plus tenacity, honesty, and a sense of humor), the main thing *your kids* are going to need is flexibility. You're going to have to let things get crazy, chaotic, and messy (e.g., dishes in the sink, missing soccer sign-ups, cereal for dinner), and they're going to have to cut you some slack. And this, as we know from parenting under even the most ideal circumstances, is not always easy.

❖ *Mothers' Wisdom* ❖

At the beginning of every school year or each time Allie starts a new class or activity, I write a note to the teacher telling them that I will try to participate and support the class as much as possible. But, given my situation, I can never make a commitment because I may not be able to follow through on it. That helps keep their expectations in line but it also means that Allie is going to have to be flexible. I won't be able to do most of the stuff the other parents do, and even when I think I can, that might not turn out to be true. That can be even harder on kids than the fact that you're sick in the first place.—Stephanie

For indeed, while you will spend lots of energy worrying about the big picture (trying to quell your children's fears and explain your prognosis in a way little ones can understand), the toughest questions may be about the little things: "Why do I have to go to Sarah's again after school?" "Why can't we go shopping?" "Why can't you drive me to the beach party?"

When my kids were in preschool, we hosted a parent-education workshop as a fund raiser. The speaker said something I'll never forget, and it applies here. She told us that, "Kids are basically self-centered until they are age seven." Subsequently, I read an article explaining that the teen years are simply a return visit to these self-centered early years.

In neither case was the "self-centered" label meant as a criticism or indictment but was offered as an explanation and a warning of sorts. Its purpose, I suppose, was to make us feel better about pushing in the sand box during the toddler years and slamming doors during puberty, but all I could think of when I learned this (and my kids were one and three at the time) was that: 1) this seemed like an eternity to wait for my kids to gain a worldview beyond who knocked over their sand castle, and 2) there would only be a few short years (say, between seven and twelve years old) when the kids' first concern would not be themselves.

Keeping this in mind may help explain why asking our kids to be flexible is such a big request.

◎   ◎   ◎

When your kids learn that you're sick, when you have the big talk, they are going to care most about how you feel and how they can help you get better faster. But as your illness drags on and in the day-to-day living that follows the initial revelation, they are going to be most aware of how your illness is affecting them.

When you can't finish the costume for the school play because you were at the doctor, she'll be devastated. You'll explain that last year's Halloween costume will do in a pinch, and offer to call her teacher to explain the change of plans. She may sulk for days and you may have to let her.

If concerns about life and death are the forest, these day-to-day things are the trees. And your most important job may be getting them to see the distinction.

❖ *Mothers' Wisdom* ❖

At first it wasn't even that big of a deal for them, kind of like an adventure, and lots of play dates. But after some time, it became a bigger deal because they wanted me to be myself again. They wanted me to do things with them, all the regular stuff. Aw, Mommy when can we do this and that, and the answer was always no. And you know at some point, they just had to accept that, although that doesn't mean they liked it.—Andrea

My MS is changing constantly and therefore so am I. I know this is hard on them because one day I might be fine but the next day might be hot and I didn't get enough sleep and I won't be able to do anything. On those days, I don't have the energy or stamina to ask them a thousand times to do something or beg them to get ready for school. Like this morning, I just got in the car and started pulling down the driveway because they obviously weren't getting the point. Some moms might have been able to stay pleasant or give in or do what needed to be done by them to get out the door all smiles. Not me. When you have MS sometimes you have to take drastic measures 'cuz kids will still be kids.—Grace

My kids know what my limits are. They know, but that doesn't always mean they remember. Their initial reaction when I can't do something or take them somewhere at that very moment may be to get angry and then sometimes I really lose it with them.—Darcy

Sometimes I just sit in the middle of the floor and cry. When my daughter keeps testing me and testing me, she has to see that she's the one who has to change her behavior to help mommy.—Melissa.

Asking Your Kids to Be Patient

Patience is flexibility's first cousin, and equally important for the kids of sick moms. Kids have to be patient when mom can't move as fast, patient when she can't make their favorite meal, patient when she's looked but cannot find the missing shoes, blouse, or DVD.

Most moms are used to moving at light-speed and kids get used to this pace. Sick moms can teach the whole family to be patient by slowing everything down. Everyone will benefit from this lesson and, in fact, most kids will enjoy the slower pace after they get used to it.

In my experience, it's like those first few days of the annual Turn off Your TV Week that I work up the courage to implement. The first day or two the kids struggle to come up with enough activities to keep themselves busy and whine that "just a little TV" will get them through the afternoon. But by Wednesday, they can barely recall how to work the remote.

I think a slower pace is actually what our kids crave, but we've "cured" them of this craving with a constant onslaught of activities, lessons, outings, and amusements. If they see you enjoying quiet time, they will too. If they see you taking naps, curling up with a good book and lingering over the morning paper, they too will find internal and individual pursuits that are satisfying. If we stop filling their every waking moment with activities, they'll stop expecting it. Then when it *is* time to do something or go somewhere it will be a real treat.

✔ TRY THIS

Talk with your kids about scaling back on their extracurricular activities. See if you can collectively cut back so that they're busy, at most, only one day after school and one day on the weekend. If you've got more than one child (and especially if mom's van is still their main mode of transportation), try to synchronize their schedules so you don't end up driving all over town when you're supposed to be home with your feet up. This will give all of you more time to relax and more time together without the constant pressure of having to squeeze too many things into too little time.

Asking Your Kids to Be Honest

In your words, actions, and reactions, you want to create an atmosphere of openness and dialogue. Be honest with your kids and ask them to be honest with you. Ask them to tell you how they're feeling, what's bothering them, and what makes them angry. Ask if they have questions about your illness that have gone unanswered. Ask them to help you come up with ways to make their "new life" with a sick mommy more like their "old life." There may be things they think you can't do that you can— and vice versa. If they know it's okay to cry, complain, and inquire when they're sad, mad, or confused, no one will have to suffer alone, or unnecessarily. When all the cards are on the table, everyone can play.

✔ TRY THIS

Start a family journal in which everyone gets to write (or scribble, sketch, or collage) their feelings about the changes going on at home. Leave it in a central location for all to pick up at will. When one person is finished, he places it back in the agreed-upon spot so it's available if someone else wants to make an entry. You may want to use the journal as a catalyst for conversation at your family meetings. Making the journal could be a family activity as well, and you don't have to exhaust yourself driving here and there to get materials for the project. A spiral notebook, some felt-tip markers, and some gift-wrapping ribbon will do the trick. You can even give the assignment to your kids and let them decorate the journal and present their master-piece at your first "meeting."

✔ AND THIS

Make sure dad (or another important adult in your kids' life) has some time alone with each of your kids each week. When you're not present, they may feel more comfortable asking some of the questions they have and it may be possible to nip some of their concerns in the bud if dad purposely sets aside time to hear them out.

Asking Your Kids to Be on the Team

In addition to being flexible, patient, and honest, your children can help in other ways as well. Dust off the job chart that's languishing on the refrigerator, reinstate the Saturday morning chore routine that has given way to just another hour of Cartoon Network, resume paying allowance or otherwise rewarding help that's above and beyond the day-to-day assignments of getting the beds made and the dirty dishes into the sink.

Just like getting used to a slower pace, kids can get used to doing more around the house to help out. So often, it's simply a matter of asking for their help. How often do you stand above a pile of just-used towels in the bathroom, and think, *The kids really should pick these up.* And how often do you just bend down and do it anyway because it will take less energy than corralling them and setting them to the task? But if you begin to set a higher bar for the kids and consistently ask them to reach it, the towels might not end up on the floor in the first place. At the very least, it should take less prodding to get them away from the GameBoy and back into the bathroom to finish the job.

As healthy moms we may have demonstrated an ability or willingness to pick up the wet towels, the dirty gym socks and the errant pieces of popcorn scattered all over the living room floor; as sick moms we cannot. And just as our health crisis may spawn a new era of closeness and communication in our homes, it may also spell an end to the era when everyone simply expects that "Mom will do it." There is no *I* in "team," as they say, but there is in "sick," and it stands for "*I* can't do it alone."

❧ *Mothers' Wisdom* ❧

You know how kids say "Mom" in just that certain way, all whiny and drawn out? Even when all they say is your name, you know they want something. There are times when I hear that from the other room, and just think, *No way, I can't do it. She's just going to have to figure it out herself.*—Paula

Today my four-year-old yelled back at me, "You're always telling me to do everything," and I just yelled back, "That's

right, and too bad, because mommy can't." It was a low
point, but he has to get it that mommy can't do everything,
even on my best days.—Grace

Use your sickness to remind everyone (including yourself)
that the family ship only sails if everyone is onboard and "all
hands are on deck." Review which chores are mandatory and
"just part of being in the family" and then invite everyone to
think of other ways they could help and post it on the hallway
closet. Maybe Susan can make dinner once a week. Maybe
Jimmy can give the dog a bath. Maybe Rachel could fold the
laundry.

It will be different for every family, but this will be a concrete
and positive way for your kids to turn their fears into action.

◎　◎　◎　◎　◎　◎　◎　◎　◎　◎　◎　◎　◎　◎　◎　◎　◎

Things You Can Do to Help When Mom Feels Tired

Moms who are sick need comfort. Doctors and daddies
do their part, and kids can do theirs by finding new
ways to spend time with mom and by helping around
the house.

Find a Quiet Activity to Do Together

- listen to music or a book on tape

- play a board game

- watch a movie together

- break out some new crayons and coloring books

- look through old photo albums

- tell stories
- paint her toenails

Help with Chores Around the House

- fold the laundry
- bring stuff up and down the stairs
- pick up your toys, clothes, and books
- bring in the mail
- feed the dog
- ask Mom or Dad what else you can do to help
- change the sheets on Mom's bed and fluff her pillows

◉ ◉ ◉ ◉ ◉ ◉ ◉ ◉ ◉ ◉ ◉ ◉ ◉ ◉ ◉ ◉ ◉

PART III

• • • • • • • •

HOW YOUR
ILLNESS AFFECTS
YOUR RELATIONSHIPS

DADDIES

Staying Together "In Sickness and In Health"

⊙　⊙　⊙　⊙　⊙　⊙　⊙　⊙　⊙　⊙　⊙　⊙　⊙　⊙　⊙　⊙　⊙

When I was young and I heard those well-known words from the marriage ceremony, I always pictured two little gray-haired people spending their twilight years together just as they had promised to do so long ago. In my mind's eye, one of the octogenarians was pushing the other in a wheelchair, or they were both walking with canes, or maybe one was visiting the other in the hospital, but they were *old* and at peace, having entered together a stage of life that is often dominated by matters relating to health. In this scenario, "sickness" kind of went with the territory—just like being exhausted goes with the being newly married with young children, and being broke goes with the stage where you're sending kids to college and saving for retirement.

As such, it really never occurred to me that our wedding vows would be tested before my husband and I had even turned forty. But they were. And it was a test we almost failed.

Indeed, the darkest days of our marriage, days when I thought our union wouldn't survive, came during this time. It seems that whoever penned the well-known promise about sticking together "in sickness and in health" knew what they were talking about.

Being sick is a strain on even the strongest marriages. Just listen to what some moms—and dads—had to say on the subject:

❖ Mothers' (and Fathers') Wisdom ❖

When Marty was diagnosed with thyroid cancer, I was stuck on the career plateau after ten years with the same company. At that stage of my life, I was in my late forties and not feeling too resilient about my professional future. Mentally, I was very preoccupied with this. However, I found it extremely difficult to share my frustrations and worries with Marty. After all, she was facing a far greater hurdle in life than I was. Obviously, I felt guilty for laboring over my work-related concerns and sensed that on occasion, I was not always emotionally there for her. In the end, we both made it through remarkably well, but I feel that I could have been more nurturing had I not been so self-absorbed at time.
—Peter S.

It was very hard to take care of all the things we normally have in our lives (especially maintaining performance at work and being there for the children) while taking on all the challenges of learning about breast cancer, helping Jennie manage her course of treatment, and being there for her at each stage of diagnosis, case review, consultations, treatment, and recovery. What a juggling act, especially since kids need someone to be there for them all the time, and even more so at times like this. It stretched me and wore me out like no other challenge I have faced.
—Rob

I expected to react more strongly but either found myself resigned to the future or needing to remain strong for others in the day. It was at night when everyone else was asleep that I felt an overwhelming despair.—Peter H.

I think the spouses get forgotten. Everyone is so sorry for you that you're sick, but nobody thinks about them. In my situation, my husband really got a raw deal. He lost his skiing buddy, his bike mate, his hiking partner. That's not what he bargained for but it's what he got. And you know what he says? He says, "It's hard on me, it's hard on Allie (our daughter), but it's hardest on you."—Stephanie

It's really hard on the spouse. You are torn up inside about what's happening to the person you love most in the world, but you are also overwhelmed by having to handle all your usual responsibilities in addition to taking over all the stuff for the kids and being there for all your wife's doctors' appointments. Everywhere you look there's someone that needs something from you and you feel selfish if you complain.—John

How You Can Keep Your Marriage Healthy Even When You're Not

The husband-wife dynamic in a family with a sick mommy is tricky on the best days and downright volatile on many others. Both partners are being asked to assume a new role in a relationship that has long operated on a fairly static set of rules and norms. And while this plays out differently with each couple, confusion about the new roles reigns and before long a dangerous combination of guilt and resentment can begin to build. For moms, you may fall into the rut of talking to your partner about nothing but test results, doctors' visits, and the logistics surrounding the kids and their activities. But when you don't share the emotional stuff, you rob yourself of a shoulder to cry on when you need it most.

Conversely, dads may retreat into the world of work where at least they understand the rules of engagement and there's a predictable pattern to most days. Moms might decide their partners shouldn't be "burdened" with the ups and downs of their medical saga or bothered with the complicated matrix you've devised to keep things running smoothly at home, choosing instead to keep these responsibilities on their own shoulders. Dad might be struggling at work or in other areas of their life but may feel it's "not the right time" to bring any of that up because their spouses are "far worse off" than they are and it would be selfish to talk about what's on their mind.

But while all these reactions are understandable, as is a craving for some semblance of normalcy, this is a scary time for everyone and no one should have to face it alone or be expected to "handle it" without help. In each other, you've got an ideal comrade and confidante. It's intimate and scary to truly share the deep emotions that illness churns up in each of you, but I suggest that risk is worth taking because the reward can be so huge— and the alternative can be so devastating.

Families are systems and all systems crave balance, homeostasis. Therefore, when mommy gets sick and the system is thrown out of balance, the shift may create profound anxiety as the family system fights to regain its old balance. If the family understands their struggle, the anxiety can be catalytic; it can be used as a wave to be ridden into all kinds of changes. Thus, the illness contains the seeds for an odd sort of gift: a paradigmatic shift that would not have occurred otherwise.

In my practice, spouses have expressed anger about what it's like to have their lives thrown upside down by their partner's illness and they feel guilty for having these feelings. Many withdraw into denial, spending more time away from home, while others are able to use the crisis as an opportunity for reflection and, ultimately, transformation. I have found that families who reach out for help—to one another, their extended families and communities—are more likely to allow the illness to have a positive effect. Often, however, people isolate. They are afraid of being seen as a burden, are ashamed of having such huge and unfamiliar needs and the system becomes even more strained."
—Valerie S. Johns, *M.A., M.F.T., adjunct professor of clinical psychology, Antioch University, Los Angeles*

What You Need To Know

◎ Understand that the usual **division of labor** in your family will be turned upside down when you're sick and you're going to have to let your husband or partner not only take care of *you* but take care of lots of other things around the house.

◎ The hardest thing of all is going to be letting this happen and **letting go of your guilt.**

◎ It's going to be clumsy, uncomfortable, and scary, but if you open up and talk about what's going on and how you're each feeling, it can bring you together rather than tear you apart. **So don't just sit there, say something!**

Role Reversal and the Division of Labor

The complicating factor when mommy becomes ill or disabled is that in most families, even the most liberated ones, mom still shoulders most of the responsibility when it comes to things related to the kids and the home. And this is true regardless of whether or not she works outside the home. So when mommy gets sick everything is thrown out of whack.

This wreaks havoc with the division of labor that has been established in the home and the method by which things get done from the mundane to the most spectacular.

If mom has to spend time in the hospital, Susie's long, fine hair might go a week without being brushed properly. She might get nothing more than a Pop-Tart for breakfast. Her lost shoes might never be found and she may go off every day in mismatched clothes and snow boots even though it hasn't snowed in weeks.

To be fair, in many cases it's not that men can't or don't want to help, it's that moms can be hesitant delegators, especially when it comes to things around the house. A lot of the details about the kids' schedules, when the gardener comes, and what day the dry cleaning will be ready are kept inside our heads. As much as dads might want to pitch in, they don't stand a chance unless we clue them in. If they want to help, that should be enough. They shouldn't have to be mind readers as well. And when we *do* let them help, we have to turn it over *and then keep our mouths shut and our hands idle.*

❧ Mothers' Wisdom ❧

The biggest mistake I have made is when I ask my husband for help and then lose patience waiting for him to do it, whatever I asked him to do. It may be cleaning the bathroom or getting the dirty dishes out of the sink, but too often he takes "too long" in my opinion and I just go ahead and do it. This happened before I got sick too but matters more now because I really should be conserving my energy, but I can't seem to ignore the muddy footprints on the floor or let the dishes sit there.—Fern

Since it doesn't really matter if there are dirty dishes in the sink, what the kids wear to school, or if they eat the occasional breakfast pastry, sick moms need to think before they speak because there's a lot more at stake than how our kids look when they leave the house and whether the house is immaculate. Nancy says it was hard to let go of the things she considered "her realm," but it became obvious that's exactly what she needed to do. (That was her daughter with the snarled hair and snow boots.)

Things were done differently, to say the least, and a lot of this stuff would have driven me crazy before, but after what we'd been through and all he'd done, I learned to keep my mouth shut, more or less.
—Nancy

Dave, Nancy's husband, could sense that letting go was hard for his wife—but he realized he really needed her to do so if he was going to truly take charge and do so without being second-guessed.

Nancy wanted to be up and about and running things. Beyond the issue of whether that would interfere with her recovery, there was my sense that I was now running the home front and I didn't want all that much input.
—Dave

Andrea learned this same important lesson while recovering from back surgery.

I made the mistake a few times but pretty soon realized that
I needed to accept the way he cooked the eggs and just be
thankful that he's bringing me food or helping with the
laundry, and not say, "That's not how the kids like them"
or "You didn't fold that right."
—Andrea

She admits, however, that her marriage was spared a lot of the
stress that might have come with her illness because she was able
to afford nine-to-five help.

Our marriage wasn't tested as much as it might have been
because we could afford help. It wasn't like Robert had to
come home to a messy house. He didn't have to deal with
the mess, do all the laundry or cook all the meals. If he'd
had to come home to that, if he'd had to do my job, that
would have been a lot harder on both of us.
—Andrea

Melissa suggests that it's not the role reversal that's hard but
the assumption of entirely new roles for *both* parties that makes
illness so hard on a marriage.

I really don't want to rely on my husband when it comes to
my disease. I want to be his wife, not his patient. I want
him to be my husband, not my nurse. But that's not
something I can always control. Sometimes I am just the
patient, the person in bed who needs everything done for
them.
—Melissa

✔ TRY THIS

One of the great things that came about after my illness, and my newly cultivated ability to let Justus parent his own way without my interference, was the initiation of "crazy days." Now whenever I am going out of town and dad's left in charge, the kids call it "crazy days." And this means, junk food, staying up late, unmade beds, mismatched clothes, etc. I watch as they stock up on supplies (chocolate doughnuts and Chips Ahoy are a must) on the days before my departure and *I keep my mouth shut*. What could be better? They're happy. I'm happy. The last thing I want to do is screw it up by delivering a lecture on nutrition, tooth decay, or why we don't wear stripes and polka dots together.

Guilt

We spoke about guilt earlier, but guilt in the domestic realm is the worst kind of all. Most moms feel guilt about being needy, guilt about not being able to take care of the kids, the laundry, the cooking, and we feel guilty that our husband's might have to miss work or their weekly golf game to care for us or the kids. For, as women (and especially mothers), we're used to getting everything done and handling whatever comes up. When we get sick we're conflicted, confused, and guilty. We want our husbands' help, we need it, but we feel guilty taking it and asking for it. It feels like a 'lose-lose' proposition.

❖ *Mothers' Wisdom* ❖

I know he felt terrible about what happened to me, but after a while I know he was tired of having other people in our house all the time helping me out and I felt guilty that I couldn't do any of the stuff I usually do. After a while, you could cut the tension with a knife. It was the worst time in our marriage.—Sue

He could always count on me before to do "my half" or more. Now all that has changed and I feel so bad about that.—Jennifer

I would bend over backwards getting friends to step in and help so that he wouldn't be bothered and he'd get upset because he'd already said he could handle it and then I robbed him of that chance to help. My guilt got the best of me and even though he said he'd do something I still felt guilty accepting that help and thought I should try and do it without him. When you're sick, everything is off balance in the family, in your relationship, and with your husband you have to withdraw so much more from the account than you put in. You may not be able to make any deposits when you're sick, but you try to withdraw less so it won't be as hard to get things back in balance once you're better.—Jennie

Just as your illness often feels like a silent, lurking force that shows you no mercy, guilt and resentment can be a "cancer" on your relationship that will render it unrecognizable if the feelings aren't shared. Based on my experience, and that of the other moms whose stories grace these pages, the only "cure" for these potentially destructive emotions is to throw open the curtains, let the sunshine in, and get everything out in the open. You've got to start talking.

Indeed, once the question was asked, the daddies in this book said loud and clear that they didn't want us to feel guilty about asking for help, they just wanted us to ask *and then accept* the help they had to give.

Don't Just Sit There, Say Something

Too often, the inner turmoil both partners are feeling during this time goes unspoken. Your husband may be feeling a confusing mixture of "Who am I to complain? She's the one who's sick, after all," (that's guilt) and "Between caring for my wife and my kids there's never a minute left over for me." (resentment).

You are probably vacillating between feeling terrible that you've had to drop the ball on almost everything you usually do—"I feel so bad just lying here all day," (guilt) and wondering why your husband isn't more like you, "I can't believe he forgot to use fabric softener and he still hasn't gone to the market" (resentment). And you too might be stressed about the work piling up on your desk while you're away.

But if no one says anything, the tension mounts and this hurts your relationship *and* your health.

As long as both of you stay in your own heads, it's unlikely that you're going to be able to move forward or get closer. For both partners, getting unstuck and getting the help and understanding you need means, as it so often does, being both a better talker and a better listener.

I didn't ask Justus to attend a single doctor's appointment, handle a single kid-related matter, or do anything extra around the house when I was sick. Then, I got resentful when he didn't and started to look for other things that were "bugging me" about our relationship, such as his long hours at work or demanding travel schedule. Because we weren't talking about what was really going on and I wasn't even remotely communicating my real needs and feelings, we had lots of big fights about lots of truly inconsequential things.

In your relationship, the lightning rod issue might be your partner's golf game, his long commute that gets him home just minutes before the kids go to bed, or his obligations to care for his aged parent, but whatever it is, it's only masking the real issue—which is the fear, confusion, and resentment that has snuck into

your marriage behind the mask of your illness and is now the big
boogeyman in the corner.

❧ *Mothers' Wisdom* ❧

I finally realized that I had to ask Danny specifically for
what I needed. For example, I needed him to remember to
ask me how I was feeling when he came home from work, to
ask about my doctors' appointments and, if I was waiting for
test results, to know when they were expected and ask me
about them when they came in. Even if this meant writing it
down in his calendar, so be it. I realized this was important
to me and he wasn't doing it consistently until I asked. When
I did finally ask he was happy to oblige.—Stephanie.

Family therapists and experts who study gender differences
would applaud Stephanie's approach. As a rule, men like specific
information about what needs to be done and how they can be of
help—and then they don't want to be second-guessed or micro-
managed. Women, often afraid of asking for what they really
need but needing it nonetheless, are frequently coy or vague
about stating their wants or desires, only to end up disappointed
because their cryptic cry for help went unheeded or was misun-
derstood.

Like everything in marriage, or any important relationship,
when you don't talk about the big things, the small things can
take on undue and disproportionate significance and can cause
big problems. For me to stop blaming Justus for the upheaval,
pain, and confusion I was feeling, I needed to take a deeper look
inside myself for the answers to the question "What am I supposed to learn from this experience?" And for me to stop resent-
ing Justus for not providing the help I needed, I had to figure out
what I needed and how to ask for it, and he had to do the same.

Most importantly, I learned that my illness was not his fault, and that my recovery was not his responsibility.

What about Sex?

When you're first sick, sex may be the furthest thing from your or your husband's mind. There's almost constant thought and talk about your body—but none of it's about how you fill out your jeans, how you look in that strapless gown, or how your perfume puts him in the mood. Most of the time, your body feels more like an old appliance that needs repair than anything remotely sensual. But as illness lingers or your recovery drags on, the issue of sex, and the larger issues of body image and intimacy, inevitably arise—and it can be devastating.

❖ *Mothers' Wisdom* ❖

It's scary to have sex when your body's been damaged and when it happens at first, you're way too scared to ask the doctors about it. It's not like in the soap operas when the doctors pronounce that the patient is ready to resume an active sex life, you're left pretty much to figure it out on your own. And for me it wasn't really about not feeling sexy, it was more that I'd just been through so much. I hate to sound like a cliché, but sometimes it really is like "Not tonight, I have a headache," but I mean a *real* headache, or some other pain that's too big to ignore.—Stephanie

When I was first diagnosed before I even had my surgery, sex was hard for me to get into the mood for. After all, who wants to have sex with a diseased woman? I found out quickly that my husband did. One of the most kind and tender things he did for me even before my operation was to touch my affected breast, feel the tumor, and tell me that it was still a part of me, even though it was cancer. After my operation we eased back into things after a few weeks. At first, I kept a T-shirt on (I had had reconstruction but was feeling self-conscious since there was no nipple). I used the T-shirt as a "transition object" for a few months afterward because it took both of us time to get used to my reconstructed breast and my abdominal scar. Then again, after chemo, I found I needed another transitional object because now I was bald, and at first I would only participate in sex if I had a hat or scarf on. But since I was the only one who seemed to care, I quit worrying about it. When I was too sick for sex because of chemo, Peter would patiently wait, not even mentioning it or indicating he would like it. Sometimes, when I was feeling better but not good enough yet for the whole thing I would remember to pleasure him. This meant a lot to him and it helped strengthen our relationship. It showed him that even though I was very ill, I had not forgotten about him.—Jennifer

This area of our relationship hasn't had any affect on [my husband]. With my disease it is mostly me who's not wanted to be intimate for whatever reason, sometimes related to my illness and sometimes not. I am now wearing a[n insulin] pump, and I sometimes feel "not pretty." But Jeff has always been a caring and compassionate person and doesn't seem to see the things that I see or feel.—Shelley

I think someone once said that [MS] is the disease of "used to be." There are just some things I can no longer do. Raising two boys and having MS is tiring, which means I'm often too tired for sex, and added to that I have loss of feeling to some degree. So the energy that it requires for me to achieve orgasm can be considerable. I guess based on Maslow's hierarchy of needs, sexual gratification is not constantly of great importance to me, but I am sad for my husband that our sex life is not hot hot hot.—Grace

During my illness itself, intercourse itself was completely out of the question. We were too busy, too concerned, too tired, and there were many times and long stretches when I was just too cut up. I knew all along, however, that my husband still found me desirable. It was because he took such good care of me—and that is its own kind of intimacy. He was attentive and affectionate and as physical as seemed appropriate. The big question, then, was when were we ready for more? I don't remember that we had a big discrepancy on this. I do remember the first time, however, being just absolutely awful because it was painful to me. I'd had abdominal surgery and I had this giant scar that had taken three months to heal, and I *felt* fine and *seemed* fine, but having an orgasm was just torture on that whole area—it pulled all the wrong places. I remember just weeping, thinking that it always would be. I said something to my surgeon, and he told me a funny story about another patient of his who claimed the same surgery had made her unable to have an orgasm, but he suspected she had a boatload of other troubles and probably never had! This was his somewhat goofy yet effective way of reassuring me that it wouldn't be bad forever. I have a fake breast, and at first I was hyperaware about my husband touching it or not touching it. He seemed almost not to notice that it wasn't real, and the one thing I really hated was when he would caress the fake breast with his mouth. I hated it because I couldn't feel it, and that was like a giant neon light flashing, "*Fake, fake.*" But I also hated it when he ignored it. I tried to tell him how I felt, but I don't think he ever really understood. My awareness has greatly diminished over time, but I have to say that this is the one time and place when I am most reminded that I lost a breast.

I guess this shouldn't be a big surprise, but it sometimes is.
—Jennie

A few other moms wanted to share about this aspect of their illness and recovery, but asked to do so anonymously:

"I can remember when I came home from the hospital. I really wanted to have sex, and that's not really like me to be so focused on that. But there was something very profound and grounding about it, scars and bandages and all."

"When I was well enough to have sex again, my husband was really caring and gentle and going very slow and I recall appreciating it for a while and then having the really strong feeling that I just wanted him to go for it and even if it hurt a little, I wanted to feel it, wanted my body to have that sensation again after all the other things it had been through. It was like declaring my independence from the doctors, from the pain, from the trauma of it all."

"I don't remember having sex much at all during the weeks and months after my recovery. I was just too freaked out about everything that happened and I think my husband thought he had to stay away and I didn't know how to break down the barrier that had built up. It's like we'd taken on new roles and sex wasn't a part of that and I didn't know how to introduce it back in."

"There are lots of times when I am not in the mood to have sex but I don't think it's fair that my husband doesn't get to have sex just because I'm sick. I know it sounds old-fashioned, but I think it's part of my wifely obligations, and if he wants it, it's the least I can do. Unless I am feeling really lousy, I try to give him this pleasure."

I can relate to many of these sentiments and I, too, was gun shy asking the doctor about sex and nervous about how my illness and recovery would affect our love life, as it would permanently alter my appearance in a fairly prominent place—right on my chest.

When conducting my pre-op interview, my surgeon told me that I could choose to have my pacemaker implanted either above my heart (roughly between my left breast and my collar bone) as is typically done or it could be tucked into and behind my left breast as some women prefer because it is less conspicuous. Then he very delicately suggested that given my "small size" it might be difficult to "hide" the pacemaker behind my breast and that the traditional placement would probably be best. So now when we are making love and I am lying flat on the bed, the bump that is the pacemaker stands out fairly prominently. I wonder how it looks to Justus and how it makes him feel about me and my body. He says he's "got other things on his mind" when we're between the sheets, but I realize I keep my eyes closed when he's caressing my breasts because the pacemaker seems intrusive and incongruous to the activity at hand. Indeed, most of the time, I don't even think about my pacemaker, but this is one time when I do.

Like moms who've survived cancer, who live with MS, or who have had any sort of surgery, I realize that others, especially our husband and kids, see the change in my physical appearance more often than I do. Justus sees my pacemaker when I'm naked, when I'm wearing a tank top, when I'm in my bathing suit. I really only see it when I look in the mirror. I wonder if he's stopped noticing or does it still remind him every time of how close he came to losing me?

Feeling Pretty

Although we wish it were not so, society places an inordinate amount of attention on appearance and puts forth a fairly narrow definition of what constitutes female beauty. As such, we women spend much of our lives obsessed with our bodies in one way or another. We're either too fat or too thin. Our boobs are too small or too big. Our hair is too curly or too straight. We have brown eyes and we wish for blue, blue and we wish for green. We get wrinkles, our breasts lose their "perk" and our hair turns gray. It never ends.

Then, in the middle of all this, we get sick. At first, we experience a welcome vacation from the tyranny of the media's portrayal of the ideal body type, because all we want from *our* body is for it to heal. What it looks like is suddenly very secondary.

But as we begin to live with our illness for a while, we realize that we want more from our bodies than for them simply not to hurt. We spend days or weeks in the hospital. We spend weeks or months being prodded, poked, and pricked as doctors struggle to diagnosis and treat our illness. And we wake up one day and realize we want to feel pretty again.

For some moms, this happens right away, for others it comes later, but it usually comes. Several of the moms I talked to could recall the exact day when they decided that being sick "didn't have to mean being ugly," as one put it.

Stephanie, who lives with the ups and downs of fibromyalgia, said she realized one day that "if I always looked as bad as I felt, I'd look terrible most of the time." So she's made a conscious choice to buy and wear "pretty, more feminine—even sexy— clothes, and not just be in my pajamas all the time."

Jennie and Jennifer both spoke of a renewed appreciation for their bodies after battling breast cancer and recovering from reconstructive surgery. Jennie told of buying sexy new lingerie, including "a great red bra," and Jennifer bragged of the "clingy dress with the plunging neckline" that she wore to her daughter's fifth birthday just weeks after her reconstructive surgery.

As for me, I haven't changed my style or bought anything radically different since I got my pacemaker—and that's my own little victory. I don't shy away from tank tops, spaghetti straps and blouses that cling even though different choices would keep my pacemaker (actually, the bump on my chest below which the pacemaker resides) out of sight.

It may not be pretty, but I refuse to let it make me feel ugly.

Getting Help

How to Know If You and Your Husband Should See a Counselor

I am a fan of professional therapy. Earlier, I recommend that you treat yourself to some form of individual counseling (or at least participation in a facilitated support group) to help process the many emotions associated with being sick. I feel just as strongly that couples can benefit from therapy to guide them through the often troubled waters that churn around your family ship when you are sick.

Even if you and he only go for one visit, unless you are extraordinarily insightful and open, you and your partner will benefit from having a safe place to talk about all the feelings that are swirling around. A wise third-party facilitator who has no stake in the outcome but wants to challenge each of you to be open and honest can be a tremendous help.

Unfortunately, it's harder and harder to find coverage for couples counseling in many health plans, but you may have success with free and low-cost services provided by the local chapters of the big national associations (American Cancer Society, the Wellness Community, National MS Foundation, etc.) and your local hospital. Many of these groups have spouse and family support groups for those whose loved ones are ill.

What If He Won't Go?

In most cases, women are more open to therapy than men, and female patients significantly outnumber men seeking help from counselors and therapists. So don't be surprised if your husband is hesitant. Here, however, is a chance to use your illness as an advantage. Even the toughest, least "touchy-feely" men will have to admit that their wives' illness has been hard on them and their relationship.

Tell him you see your illness as a turning point in your relationship and that while you know something about how it's affecting you, you want to know how it has affected him. Just ask him to give it a try. If he still refuses, ask if he'd consider going on his own. If he still resists, go ahead and go alone. Ultimately, you're only responsible for your own emotions.

If you're going and he's not, beware of one big mistake. Don't think that you can go for both of you. Too many times, before and after we went as a couple, I would come home from therapy and "share" all my insights with him. This conversation always went rapidly downhill. Out of context and out of the safety zone that is the therapist's office, the words spoken there and the advice rendered and repeated simply sounded like more demands from me. After all, the therapist only hears "one side of the story" and would be hard-pressed to read your partner's mind.

Should My Husband and I See the Same Counselor?

Different counselors have different opinions about this, so it may take care of itself. Also, some therapists specialize in couples therapy. However, if you have seen, or are seeing, someone on your own, your husband might feel that you'll "gang up" on him in a joint session. His resistance to going may lessen if you suggest a new, "neutral" person. He might also like to be seen by a male therapist and you may be more comfortable with a woman.

◎　　◎　　◎

I may never know the true impact on my husband of my brush with death. Guys are like that. Even my husband, who's a good communicator and very sensitive, isn't big on rehashing the past, opening old wounds, and pondering the meaning of life based on things that have happened. He's more interested in living in the present and planning for the future. He looks forward, not back. And that's fine because, as is often the case with married couples, his approach complements mine. And today, I am happy to report, the storms we survived are part of the proud lore of our marriage.

Whatever your relationship looked like before you got sick, it won't look the same after. Illness is like an uninvited houseguest or a remodeling project that is dragging on and on. Everyone in the family is affected and you and your partner better come up with a plan to manage the situation or you'll be at each other's throats.

When you're forced into new roles, your marriage will be tested, but if you really mine the experience for all it's worth, your marriage can not only survive but thrive.

What Mommies Should Know that Daddies Are Thinking

Moms should know that, barring unnatural disasters, their husbands believe—and hope—that they are fully capable of handling the situation until proven otherwise. They should also have confidence that both their spouses and their offspring are more resilient than perhaps they may think and they should relax and get well.—Dave

Like the patient, there is a whirlwind of thoughts going through a husband's mind, about everything happening in the moment, and of course concerns about the future. It is also one of the few moments when many of a person's or couples' future dreams are immediately put at risk. I think a major illness at a younger age forces many couples to face their own frailty and mortality at a stage of life when few of their peers are facing those issues and you weren't expecting to.—Rob

They should know that we are doing our best but don't always know what to do next. It's especially hard because of work pressures, and although those are very real for you, you feel like they're trivial compared to what's happening at home, and this is a difficult balancing act.—Peter S.

We're thinking about them and their illness all the time. Not that it's the only thing we're thinking of but that we're thinking of how they're doing and what we can do to help them, alleviate their pain if we can, do things that will make their lives easier. And if we aren't doing it or are doing it wrong, tell us, because we want to get it right.—Danny

It sounds kind of funny to say this out loud, to say it after everything that happened, but I wish she'd told me more that I was a good husband. I think guys need that kind of reassurance.—John

Advice for Dads from Dads

To other dads, I would say: Take advice when you need it, stay subordinated to the task at hand, admit at least to yourself that you don't know everything, remember that your wife is probably having as hard a time giving up the reins as you might if you were asked to turn your job over to somebody else, stay cool when the kids say "But Mom always . . ." Don't let any of these concerns/issues/pinpricks intrude on the main job, which is maintaining an even keel and letting the family flourish while/so that Mom gets well.—Dave

Your wife doesn't need for you to solve the problem or fully and impartially understand the disease. She needs you to be there, to listen, to hold her, reassure her, and to participate in the healing process.—Peter H.

If you married the right woman, you'll get through it. My advice would be to ensure you are doing a few basic things to take care of yourself (adequate sleep, staying in touch with friends, doing a few of the key things that help you feel good. For me, it was continuing to do a little exercise on a regular basis).—Rob

Don't think that you can't do this. You can. You can figure out about the shopping, the laundry, even how to do your daughter's hair.—John

You've got to get over it. What I mean is, get over wishing for how it used to be and how you might want it to be and focus on what *is*. What *is* is that your wife is sick and if you love her, you have to move out of denial as fast as possible and figure out what you can do that's going to help. You can't cure her, but what can you do? Pick up the dirty socks and the dog toys, bring her a cup of tea, let her rest, and get the kids to pitch in too.—Danny

GRANDMAS

Why Mommies Need Mommies
(*and Others They Can Count On*)

❀ ❀ ❀ ❀ ❀ ❀ ❀ ❀ ❀ ❀ ❀ ❀ ❀ ❀ ❀ ❀ ❀ ❀

After the birth of each of my kids, my mom came up to stay with us. At the time, we were living in a nine-hundred-square-foot, one-bedroom condo, which meant grandma was on the futon in the front room and we rolled the bassinet around from room to room (kitchen, hallway, bedroom) depending on who was home, who needed to sleep, and whether the gardener was out front using the leaf blower. We were bleary-eyed and stepping all over each other and stacks of diapers, dirty laundry, and every caring-for-your-newborn book on the market, but no one minded. We needed the help and my mom certainly couldn't imagine being anywhere else.

This is so funny in retrospect because I remember a friend (already a mom) advising me to have my mom come after the baby was born and thinking, *What is she going to do all day?* Of course once the babies came, it quickly became apparent that I couldn't do it without her—or at least I was glad I didn't have to try.

Having a baby is a life-changing experience. It is exhilarating, but it's also exhausting, overwhelming, and petrifying. You need your mommy.

The same can be said for the experience of being a sick mom—minus the exhilarating and exciting part. You are exhausted. You are scared. You can't take care of yourself or your kids (at least not the way you usually do) and there's really no one who can tend to you and take over like your mom. Even in situations where you'd say your relationship is less than ideal, having your mom around can be the best thing to ease your mind, diminish your workload, and reduce your guilt.

And in most cases, you're not even going to have to ask. Because moms are programmed to know what their kids need and take care of it—even when the "kid" is you.

No Way, Not My Mom!

Not every mother/daughter relationship will be able to weather this storm and come out stronger. If you know that ahead of time, don't ask the relationship to be something it cannot. Unrealistic expectations or the belief that a previously testy relationship will be made whole through your illness can add to tremendous stress and distract you from the only job that really matters, which is to work on getting better. Maybe your mom isn't the one to move in and help you with the cleaning, cooking, and laundry. But maybe she can order your Christmas cards or take the kids back-to-school shopping. Maybe you don't want your mom accompanying you to doctors' appointments. But she may be the perfect one to run an errand to the pharmacy or surprise you with a thick new bathrobe from the Eddie Bauer catalog. Then again, your mother's fear and sadness about your illness may paralyze her and render her totally useless or find her involving herself in your life in all the wrong ways.

Said one sick mom, "I got so exhausted trying to do all the things my mom suggested and follow up on all the advice and tips she was gathering for me when all I really wanted was for her to come sit on the floor and play with the kids and hold my hand. But, I learned, that's not who my mom is and I finally just had to accept that. I accepted that she wasn't going to be there for me like I needed, but I also stopped trying to please her by trying to fight my illness her way. It was sad but kind of freeing to let this go."

When mother-daughter relationships are working well, it's often because your mom knows what you need before you've even asked. With other people, even your husband, there can be some anxiety about asking for help in the first place (so much so that we often don't do it) and then guilt when we *do* ask and the help arrives. But letting your mom take the kids on an outing, cook your dinner, or fold the laundry is a great way to get some rest and practice asking for and receiving help without feeling that you're then going to have to return the favor.

Why Mommies
Need Mommies

◉ If your mom has offered to come, let her. If she hasn't offered, ask her to. In most cases, this will be the easiest way to get the help you need—and there should be no guilt or feeling that you need to reciprocate. This is simply *what moms do*. You know that, you do it for your kids every day.

◉ Even if you and your mom don't always get along and you feel like she's always critiquing you, call for a truce or simply ignore this so you can have another set of eyes and hands in the house to watch the kids and wash the dishes.

⊚ Your illness and your ability to let your mom serve you in this way may open a new chapter in your relationship and this may be one of the very positive lasting effects of this crisis.

⊚ Even though you're letting her help you, it's still your house, and to the degree you care (and have energy to worry about it), you can ask your mom to adhere to certain rules with the kids or to follow certain procedures around the house.

⊚ Just don't forget that the kids can survive ice cream for lunch, TV during dinner, and even missed homework assignments if it means you're resting and preparing for the day when you can return to the kitchen, the car pool, and the homework "help" desk.

A Few Words for Moms without Moms

For some women, having your mother help out when you're sick may simply not be an option. You may have determined, as discussed above, that it's unrealistic to expect your mom to help in the way you'd like or need. And even if she *is* the person you'd most like to have at your bedside, your mother may live in a distant city on a limited income, work full-time, or have passed away. For these mommies, it's good to look at what characteristics can make grandmothers such an ideal helper and see who else might fit the bill. It might be your dad, your aunt, your sister, a neighbor, or a friend. These are the characteristics as I see them:

⊚ someone who loves you and knows you well

⊚ someone with few binding obligations (if it's a friend, it helps if he/she doesn't have young kids living at home) so that he/she might even be able to come and stay with you while you heal

⊚ someone you wouldn't mind seeing you with your house a mess, your hair dirty, and your laundry piled high

⊚ someone you can ask for help without feeling the need to reciprocate or write a thank-you note

As we've discussed throughout, you are going to need a whole cadre of helpers, people who you can call at the drop of a hat, people who simply show up with a smoothie at just the right moment. The great thing about grandma (or another person of her ilk) is that she's in your life to stay and she'll do anything for you, no questions asked and no thank-you necessary.

It's easiest to get this concept when you imagine one of your own kids getting sick. No matter their age, no matter their circumstances, you'd drop everything and then do anything you could to lighten their load and speed their healing. That's what she can do for you. That's why mommies need mommies.

Listen to
Your Mother

My mom may not have coined any of these sayings, but I heard them first from her and they have become my favorite mantras:

⊚ Wear it like a loose garment (in other words, "Hang loose").

◉ Wisdom is holding two opposing views at the same time.

◉ God's timing is always perfect.

◉ Take it fifteen minutes at a time.

◉ Just dry the teacup (as in, "Do one thing at a time").

GIRLFRIENDS

Defining and Redefining What You Need from Your Friends

◎ ◎ ◎ ◎ ◎ ◎ ◎ ◎ ◎ ◎ ◎ ◎ ◎ ◎ ◎ ◎ ◎ ◎

Friendships, especially females ones, change dramatically during the course of our lives. What we need from our friends is dictated by our stage in life and we seek out different people at different times.

When we're young we need playmates and confidantes—and this is true, to a certain extent, from the time we're about eight until whenever we get married or seriously attached to a boyfriend or partner. The way we "play" and the things we like to do may change, but we're usually looking for someone to play *with*, friends who share our interests and concerns. Later when we're married or dating, our single girlfriends take a backseat role, as we find ourselves drawn to other women in committed relationships with husbands or boyfriends we (and our partner) like and we commence with double dating, ski weekends, and intimate dinner parties.

Then we become mothers.

For a while, we're so tired we don't even miss our old life.

We just crave sleep. Then as the exhaustion begins to wane, we find ourselves seeking out other moms with babies and pepper each other with questions about diaper rash, thumb sucking, and whether our children will ever sleep through the night. Our friends become other moms because they're the only ones who "really get it." You still have college friends, work friends, maybe even childhood chums, but your best friends are often those who are going through what you're going through at the same time.

So what happens when you get sick? Do we now have to seek out another group of sick friends? That sounds pretty depressing.

Well, the answer is yes and no.

We find when we're sick that other women who've been through what we're going through, especially those who've battled the same disease, can be a great comfort. They don't have to ask a lot of the basic questions that may irritate us when we've already had to answer them a hundred times responding to well-meaning questions from our "well" friends. They'll probably be able to anticipate some of your needs before you even open your mouth. They may be able to compare medical notes and refer you to doctors, clinics, or other resources that may be of value. Moms who've been sick understand what moms who are sick need. Their support is invaluable.

But you don't want to talk only of your illness, receive only visitors bearing casseroles, or live in a world devoid of idle chat and lighthearted news about the girls' soccer team, the school's new math teacher or who was wearing what at last week's dinner dance. Just because being sick is serious business doesn't mean you have to be serious all the time.

Your friends might feel it's frivolous to talk to you about things that are "so insignificant compared to what you're going through," but you crave such banter. Because they may feel it's inappropriate to talk about "the regular stuff," you may have to specifically ask for it. It's an invitation to gossip. Everyone's wondering how he or she can help; here's another answer.

When your friend from temple asks what she can do, tell her you want to know everything about what's been happening since your longtime and popular rabbi announced she was leaving. When the mother of your son's best friend calls, ask her to regale you with details about the baseball team's annual barbeque and awards banquet. When your pal from work drops by, tell her you want to know the latest about the supposed tryst going on between the guy in marketing and the gal in personnel.

It doesn't matter what you talk about—as long as it's not about your illness. Sure, they'll want to know how you're feeling and what's the latest news from the doctor and you can tell them, but make it clear that you feel cut off from the normal routine and that simply talking is a great way to help keep you plugged in and give you something else to think about. It's like getting a copy of *People* magazine when all you've been reading is the *Harvard Business Review* or the *New England Journal of Medicine*. Your illness hasn't robbed you of the desire to laugh and have fun. Maybe you can't *do* all the things you used to do, that doesn't mean you don't want to talk about it.

❖ *Mothers' Wisdom* ❖

It's not like I missed going out with girlfriends or spending big chunks of time with girlfriends, because I didn't really do that *before* I was sick. What I missed, though, was all the little stuff. I missed dropping the kids off at school, because waving at moms in the other cars and chatting for two minutes at the curb was where my friendships happened. After a while, I was just craving the dumbest comments—new lipstick stories, ornery kid stories, anything but cancer.—Jennie

PAYCHECKS

Balancing Work and Recovery

❀ ❀ ❀ ❀ ❀ ❀ ❀ ❀ ❀ ❀ ❀ ❀ ❀ ❀ ❀ ❀ ❀

B eing a sick mom is hard.
Being a sick working mom is even harder.

And while we all agree that every mom is a "working mom," for those who have to get up and go to the office or spend their day in front of the computer at home, there is an extra burden. And like everything related to being a working mother, the pressures are both monetary and personal as you seek to contribute financial resources to your family *and* chart a course for yourself professionally in spite of (and sometimes, because of) having a family to raise.

The good news is work gives us another place to practice asking for help, saying no and testing what our priorities really are in the face of a world turned upside down by illness. It's my belief that being sick can even improve a mother's delicate work/family balance as she may be forced to make concessions or adjustments at work that she never would have considered before. Having done so, she can step back and analyze what role she wants (or needs) work to play in her life.

That was Catherine's experience.

Educated and trained as an attorney, Catherine has made numerous career decisions based on her diabetes diagnosis, which came a few days before her thirty-second birthday.

At the time, I had no health insurance so I accepted a job at two-thirds of my current salary just to get those benefits. The work and office environment were miserable but cushioned me long enough to get my head around the diagnosis and the day-to-day management of my illness. Finally, I left for a better salary and more challenging work. Well, "challenging" was the word for it. My new job (as a union representative) included a seventy-mile commute each way in addition to driving while on the job. That created a whole new wrinkle in managing my insulin injections.

My boss was aware of my illness but lacked the courage to work with me creatively on solutions. I proposed working from my home office once or twice a week, but he refused. The last straw, I guess for both of us, was when I had a severe hypoglycemic episode on the eve of an important arbitration. The paramedics had to come in the middle of the night. It was the first time I had required assistance in raising my blood sugar levels and it was terrifying.

I had to cancel the arbitration and my boss used that as an excuse for the growing rift between us. I was alienated from colleagues at work and under scrutiny by support staff that had been tasked by my boss with monitoring my health and activities. The whole situation became intolerable.

This is also when I got pregnant for the first time and managing pregnancy and diabetes is serious business. All this contributed to my decision to quit and start freelancing.

After my first son was born, and several projects wound down, my need for regular work increased and I went job hunting again.

I had a friend at the (PR) agency and so I knew about the climate in advance, which lessened my apprehension somewhat about how I'd manage the work/health/family balance. A few months after starting at the agency, I discovered that I was pregnant again. And because of my illness and complications at the end of my first pregnancy, I was in and out of the doctor's all the time and even monitored three times a week during my last trimester.

Well, my candor with everyone at work paid off, confirming I was in the right place. My boss and the entire agency worked with me to craft an appropriate leave even though I hadn't really been there long enough to accumulate the time and they never made me feel as though my position was in jeopardy because of my diabetes, my pregnancy, or my family.
—Catherine

While every sick working mother's experience is different, Catherine's example of putting her needs first—and continually reexamining them—reminds us that jobs and bosses will come and go but the need to safeguard our health is constant.

◉   ◉   ◉

Catherine's story also highlights many of the questions faced by sick working moms, the answers to which are never easy and are always unique to each woman's situation. They include:

◉   Should I talk about my illness at work?

◉   If so, who do I tell and how much?

◉   How much time should I take off?

◉ How do I protect my job?

◉ What about resentful colleagues and angry bosses?

◉ Can I work from home when I'm sick?

◉ Should I quit or look for something different?

Deciding Whether or Not to Talk about Your Illness

The answer to the question of whether to "go public" with news of your illness at work, which is the question from which all the others flow, is governed by a whole host of factors, some in your control and some not. But, generally speaking, being free to speak candidly about your condition is highly preferable to having to hide it.

Keeping secrets and covering things up takes energy, and sick moms don't typically have any energy to spare. In addition, if you can talk about your illness at work, you might just find that you have more support and resources and people ready to pitch in than you ever knew.

That said, talking about your illness does have its risks and you have to gauge your boss, colleagues, and family financial situation in order to assess that risk. You should also consult your human resources manager or an employment attorney if you have any concerns about how your employer might react to your illness. Federal laws such as the Family and Medical Leave Act provide for time off and other protections for sick employees and those caring for them. (*Note:* The law granting twelve weeks off for full-time employees only applies to companies that "regularly employ" more than fifty people, however, some smaller companies have chosen to participate as well. Vast information about this and other pertinent regulations can be found on the Internet.

Two sites you may want to check out are: www.lawguru.com and www.employer-employee.com.)

Catherine agrees that in a best-case scenario you'll be able to talk about your condition at work. However, she cautions, "there are enlightened employers and not-so-enlightened employers. You may not know which you have and you should proceed slowly as you try to determine that." She also points out that employers, "because of their own hang-ups, prejudices, and what they do or don't know about a certain disease, may react differently to the news depending on what your particular condition is."

Fern, who has four kids and holds a prestigious position at a major state university, assessed her situation and decided she could not tell anyone at work about her cancer.

> *There have been significant layoffs here and anyone who's seen as being less than 110 percent productive could find themselves out of a job. I'm also two years away from retiring and those benefits are tremendous and would be a real help to the family. When I had my hysterectomy I had to miss a month and I had to tell them about that, but I did not tell them it was because of cancer. I've been lucky that I haven't lost all my hair during the chemo. I can just pull it back and you really can't tell. The main thing is that I've lost a lot of weight and people comment on that. But as long as I don't talk about it and I don't miss a beat at work, I think my job is safe.*
> —Fern

Nancy, a freelance writer and mother of two, recently survived two bouts of pneumonia and a pulmonary embolism. She says sick moms who work from home have an advantage since they don't have to show up every day at an office looking and acting a certain way even if they don't feel good. But, she says, don't be fooled into thinking that means illness doesn't affect your work.

> *Freelancing is a tough field and I'd be happier if most of the folks for whom I write and do research didn't think of me as ill. I pride myself on my professionalism and don't want editors having even the slightest concern about whether I might get sick and miss a deadline. I'm constantly aware that there are thousands of people who'd love to write that article if I turn it down or take on a client to whom I say no. I took off about a month, but even then I tried to keep up with my e-mail so clients would assume I was working away as normal.*
> —Nancy

Who to Tell and What to Expect

Even if you choose not to tell your boss, colleagues, or those who report to you, you should be able to safely seek out the support and counsel of your company's HR department. You'll want to understand as much as you can about your medical and disability benefits and whether, for example, vacation days can be used as part of a medical leave. You'll need to know what your employer's policy is regarding taking time off for doctors' appointments and other matters, as well. Like doctors and lawyers, human resource and employee assistance personnel are ethically bound to keep your matter private and confidential, although some are more discreet than others. Your knowledge and instincts about how the company has handled these matters in the past should inform your decision.

Some women choose to tell their boss but keep the matter from those who work for them. Some do just the opposite. Some choose only to tell a few trustworthy friend/colleagues. This is a very personal decision that can have many different outcomes. Talk with your husband and thoroughly consider all your options and the optimal outcome before deciding what to do.

Calling in Sick

With some women and some conditions, there is no choice but to tell your boss or colleagues about your illness—you're just too sick to go to work. Having come to terms with this reality, the question then arises, how much time should you take off?

First and foremost, this is a decision that needs to be made in concert with your doctor. You may need to ask this question very specifically because you may be pushed (or you may push yourself) back to work before it's safe. The proverbial "doctors' note" of your elementary school days may be just what's needed here if you need help in getting the time off you need. So ask your doctor directly, "How long should I wait before going back to full-time work?" Ask about working from home, sitting at the computer, traveling for business, taking calls, and checking e-mail. These are not silly questions, these are the things you are going to have to decide, and it's better to get your doctor's input before you get that first call from the office asking, "When can we expect you back?" You can't trust even the greatest boss to put your needs before the company's indefinitely, and you may not be able to trust yourself unless you get these questions answered. So ask the questions—and then do as you're told.

If your family situation dictates a speedy return to work and earning, try to think creatively about how you might do your job from home or on a reduced schedule, and ask your doctor specific questions like, "I think I am going to need to go back to work in about two weeks, how many hours per day would it be safe to work?" Ask if you need to limit your driving (medication may be an issue here) and, if your job includes travel, when it will be safe for you to fly.

Predicting Reactions and Protecting Your Job

While keeping news of your illness private can be exhausting, sharing the news brings challenges as well. Often when sick moms *do* tell their bosses and colleagues about what's going on, they then spend significant energy trying to make sure that no one thinks they're using their illness as an "excuse" to not perform at their usual level, and they rush back to work often before it's time.

That's what happened to me.

When I got sick, I had been at my job for about eight months. I had been hired away from an affiliated organization with the promise of a significant pay increase and promotion. I went from being a middle manager at a $3 million nonprofit to the number-two person at a $60 million foundation.

As the person responsible for the firm's strategic planning, business development, and marketing, I was in the hot seat as we sought ways to invest in the community's health (our mission) while also generating income so we could build our endowment and continue this work into the future. I was developing business plans, building collaborative partnerships, and researching new approaches for generating revenue. I had never done anything like this before. But I had lots of energy and ideas and my boss believed in me.

Needless to say, there was a lot of stress (wanting to do a good job, not wanting to let my boss down, wanting to live up to his high expectations) and I was unable to make my health a priority—even though our organization promoted programs that did just that in the community. My boss had survived several of his own health scares and talked a lot about promoting a balanced approach to work and family (and in many ways followed up this talk with concrete action), but *he* was always at the office and it was easy to feel that you weren't contributing at the expected high level.

To be fair, my overworking and the related stress had more to do with my insecurities and lack of boundaries than any dictum laid down by my employer.

No one said I had to postpone doctors' appointments in order to make a meeting, go ahead with a big presentation just hours after my MRI, or meet my boss for lunch just days after my surgery to "go over some important things" that had happened at the office in my absence.

This was all my own doing. I was the go-to person on all these projects and it unnerved me to think that someone else would step into that void in my absence. Plus, my boss treated me as if I was indispensable—and I began to believe it.

But it wasn't good for me.

Much like the pumpkin patch, the trips to the market that cheated me out of all those casseroles, and checking voice mail from my hospital bed, my return to work and everything-is-fine charade was driven by habit and fear, not conscious choice. And that's what made it so damaging.

When we fail to see life's choices, we put ourselves in a box from which there seems to be no escape. Working moms seem especially susceptible to this kind of thinking, often at great peril to their health.

⊗　　⊗　　⊗

One friend shared with me the story of her mom, who had cancer when she was growing up. "She went to chemo on Friday afternoons so she could recuperate over the weekend and be back at work on Monday and keep driving us to school, dance classes, making our dinner every night. She never wanted her illness to burden us or her coworkers. That was her main concern."

Another shared that most of her illness and recovery happened in the fall "during the holidays when people aren't working that much anyway and are pretty distracted, so it didn't really have to upset my work life very much and that was very important to me."

Still another said she chose a less invasive procedure than the hysterectomy that initially was recommended for her early-stage uterine cancer "because they said they could do it on a Thursday and I could be back at work on Monday and only miss two days. I didn't have time for the other procedure; I needed something that would fit into my schedule." Unfortunately, one year later she had full-blown cancer, had to then have the hysterectomy, rounds of chemo, and she's still not out of the woods.

❦ ❦ ❦

If this book does nothing else, I hope that it introduces the concept of choice into mothers' lives, especially sick moms. On its face, a decision to keep up appearances and productivity at work may be a good one. The problem is when we do it without thinking.

Marty, who runs her own land-use planning company, has two kids, and has battled thyroid cancer two times in the last six years, says the choices are hard—but worth making.

The first time I was sick, my kids were twelve and fifteen and my business was truly a one-woman operation. That made it hard but I chose to keep working and make it as seamless as possible for my clients because I wanted to have my business when all this was over. The second time my kids and my business had grown, which meant in both cases, less pressure on me because the kids were more or less on

their own and I had some support staff answering phones at
the office and working on bigger projects with lots of other
consultants. I am glad I have made the choices I have made.
I thought about quitting both times and decided to stick
with it.
—Marty

Unlike Marty, I was on autopilot and don't remember thinking I had any choice but to keep going full-speed ahead and try
to make up for lost time. I'm not sure that a different approach
would have had much impact on my physical health (once the
condition was diagnosed and the pacemaker implanted) but I
know it would have lessened the emotional toll the ordeal had on
my family and me.

Working mothers are used to the tug and pull their decision to
work exerts on them and their families. Even after the decision
has been made there are daily ramifications, both negative and
positive, from our choice. And this was before we got sick. When
a working mom gets sick, further strain is placed on the delicate
balance we strive for at work, and home. Decisions about who,
how, when (and *whether*) to tell your employer or colleagues
about your illness will depend on many factors, some having to
do with your illness, some having to do with your bank account,
and some relating to your relationship with your boss, clients,
colleagues, and the company's corporate culture.

But regardless of these many distinctions, one thing remains
true—your goal should be to reduce the stress and worry that
emanate from this sphere of your life. Whatever your condition,
we know it will be made worse if you are missing deadlines and
fumbling for excuses to explain your absence at key meetings. In
some cases, the path of least stress is going to be full disclosure.
In other cases it is going to be keeping the entire matter private.
Only you can be the judge. But you must promise yourself that

you'll put *your* best interest at the top of page when you begin to list the pros and cons associated with each choice.

Finally, some moms find that their illness serves as a "break in the action" from their previous go-go existence. You may come out of it with an altered sense of the place you want your work to occupy in your life, and new ideas about what might constitute a satisfying professional life. Not every working mom is going to have a choice about whether to cut back or quit working outside the home once her condition is stabilized, but some may uncover options where they once thought none existed. This too is highly personal, but if your illness has piqued in you an interest to explore other options when it comes to your career, I encourage you to explore these feelings with your husband or other close friend. Try to assess the various needs (financial, personal satisfaction, role modeling for your children, etc.) you are trying to meet through your professional endeavors and then think broadly about the many different ways you can accomplish those same goals.

Remember that, while important, none of these decisions are irreversible. To prove that, look at the many ways I have adapted my work life since the time of my illness. In the matter of just a few years, I have:

- ⊚ returned to full-time work at my original employer

- ⊚ cut my schedule to four days per week

- ⊚ cut my schedule to three days per week

- ⊚ quit to stay home full-time with my kids

- ⊚ worked ten hours per week freelancing

- ⊚ opened my own business and increased my hours to twenty-five to thirty hours per week (which corresponds with the hours my kids are in school)

Note: After accounting for taxes, day care, and the prorated three-day-a-week salary I was earning at my last job, my husband and I determined that I was netting about $20,000 annually. Once we figured that out, we looked for other ways for me to bring in that money (or more). Having a sense of that bottom-line goal freed us up to consider a lot of different options.

CAN YOU HEAR ME NOW?

Your Illness and Your Relationship (or Not) with God

⊙ ⊙ ⊙ ⊙ ⊙ ⊙ ⊙ ⊙ ⊙ ⊙ ⊙ ⊙ ⊙ ⊙ ⊙ ⊙ ⊙

When I was little, I remember being told that we shouldn't just pray when we want something but for other reasons and at other times as well. Pray for others, pray for forgiveness, pray in thanksgiving. After that, we were told, we could pray for ourselves.

This came to me in the hospital the night before my surgery when I was very *busy* praying for myself and hoped that God would forgive my lack of contact over the previous few years. I'd always had what I considered a fairly spiritual approach to life (do unto others, love they neighbor, give thanks), but I hadn't been to church in years and couldn't remember the last time I'd said more than a quick grace before dinner. But I fervently hoped that He/She/It would now be there for me in my hour of need.

It's true what they say—nothing gets you talking to God like a crisis.

When things are going well, it's easy to believe that it's all our own doing, but when the you-know-what hits the fan, many of us grab the hot line in an attempt to reach the man/woman/spirit upstairs. For others, it is a journey inside, to reach the small, intuitive voice that so often gets drowned out in the noise and bustle of everyday life.

Either way, it comes as little surprise that many mommies light candles, burn incense, get down on their knees, or sit quietly in the lotus position when they're struck with a debilitating illness and looking for answers to some of life's toughest questions.

At first, the dialogue can be rather abrupt and sounds more like a child's protestations than a saint's entreaty. "Why me!?" "It's not fair!" "Where did You go?" "What did I do to deserve this?"

But that's okay.

The conversation has begun.

Now, the tricky part about praying or meditating is not usually the talking or the thinking. It's the listening. We can state the question loud and clear, but we have to really pay attention if we're going to hear the response. In my mind, that's really the point of worship services or religious rituals of any kind. They physically remove us from our usual circumstances and put us in a place where the only activity is listening to God—or to the sound of our own breath.

When we're sick, however, it may be hard to get to the temple, shrine, church, or mosque. But we can do the same thing right in our front room, sitting in our garden, or simply lying in bed. For if you believe that a higher power is at work in your life and that your illness is part of some larger plan, you'll want to listen up and find out what the plan is. If there's a lesson to be learned, it's best to be present when the teacher speaks.

From a purely human perspective, the goal when you are sick is to be healed so you can "get on with life," so life can be about life again and not illness. That would be the perspective most people would have and they will shop

*around for the modality that works best to bring them that
healing, starting with allopathic (traditional) medicine and
then maybe moving to alternative modalities such as
acupuncture, chiropractic, herbs, etc. And the more
desperate they become, the more "far out" approaches they
are willing to try. Someone coming from this perspective
will define healing as remission of symptoms on the physical
realm.*

*But if you look at your illness from a spiritual
dimension, the question becomes, "What purpose does this
illness serve in my life?" and "What opportunity is
presenting itself for me to learn from this?" If you believe,
as I do, that we are not humans with souls but souls having
a human experience, you will see this body for what it is—
a vehicle in which to be on this earth learning the lessons
designed specifically for you in this lifetime. From a
spiritual context, there are no bad things, no right or wrong.
It's all about lessons and experiences, choices and
consequences. Seen in this light, your soul will just as easily
involve you in cancer as it will a common cold. It merely
presents you with the experiences you need to learn the
lessons you are here to learn.*

*Spirituality is about perspective and so with illness or
any other difficult thing, it's all about from what altitude
you can view the whole thing that is happening and look for
its meaning and purpose. If you're able to look at it this
way, your illness has the potential to be the most important
thing that happens in your life.*

—Ron Hulnick, Ph.D., *president of the University of Santa
Monica, a center for the study and practice of spiritual
psychology*

Whether you call it prayer, meditation, visualizing, or just
thinking, I urge you to create some space for yourself and some

quiet so that you can connect with your conscience, your inner voice, your source of strength. Sick moms need lots of help from lots of sources—not the least of which is a source that is divine, all-knowing, and all-loving. Whatever you call it, wherever you find it, I encourage you to tap into what Albert Einstein called "the illimitable superior spirit." Think of it as your quest for Jiminy Cricket—the little voice that, when listened to, has much to teach and much to offer.

> *There are three things that can happen to sick people with regards to their spirituality. One, a person may draw closer than ever and lean harder than ever on their faith tradition. Two, they may lose their faith altogether, feel further away from God than ever, or be just plain angry at God. Finally, they may want to avoid the subject entirely. And the only road family and friends can walk down in supporting the patient is the one that is open. Which means following their lead, talking and praying with them if that is what they want, or staying completely away from the subject if that is their desire. So it doesn't matter if the visitor or family member is religious or an atheist, as their friend your job is to support their beliefs.*
>
> *Indeed, religion comes from the Latin word,* religio, *which means "reconnect." So the greatest comfort of religion is that it reconnects a person to a source of strength both within and outside themselves—and this can come in as many forms as there are people, so be open to it and supportive of it.*
>
> —Jacquelin Gorman, *minister of pastoral care and hospital chaplain intern, UCLA Medical Center*

White Light

Like most people, I've heard the tales of those who nearly died and what they saw "on the other side" before they were resuscitated. They speak of white lights, encounters with Jesus, angels and other heavenly beings. They tell of floating above their bodies and watching in peaceful detachment as they pass from one state to another. Well, none of this happened to me when my heart stopped. And that frightened me.

Indeed, my near-death experience was entirely different. Not only did I miss out on the bliss, floating, and peacefulness described in the pages of *Reader's Digest,* the time I spent fighting for my life was just that—a fight. A dark, scary, cold, and noisy struggle.

My immediate concern that morning in the hospital had been trying to understand the medical aspects of my problem and the remedy that was being proposed. I was in such a state of shock that it was a few days before I began to wonder and worry about what had happened during the time my heart had stopped. Where was the "long hallway with the beacon at the end?" Where was God? Why didn't He appear and why was it so dark and scary?

Then other people started to inquire.

"Did you see the white light?" they'd ask after hearing that I had almost died during the test.

"No," I'd confess simply.

I only told a few people what I *did* see, what I *did* feel.

And I asked myself: Did this mean I was going to hell? Was that the devil? Did this mean I would never see God?

I felt so betrayed.

I'd been a good girl. I'd gone through something terrifying, and God had left me high and dry. If all this was supposed to be part of some bigger plan, why wasn't He appearing to reveal that to me?

But, God moves in mysterious ways and She would show Herself to me again and again during this crisis and its aftermath—just not in the way that sells movie tickets or magazine subscriptions. God didn't appear in a burning bush or flash of light but began to appear in the way he usually does—in the words and actions of people around me.

> *Often, people lose their faith when they get ill, especially when they are young and the illness doesn't seem "fair." They feel abandoned or punished by God.*
>
> *One therapeutic benefit that may result from a loss of faith occurs when the sufferers can come to terms with a different kind of God. If they can give up the idea that the illness is their fault, that they are being punished, that they have fallen out of grace, then they have an opportunity for a vital spiritual experience.*
>
> *I try to help my patients to understand that God doesn't dole out illnesses based on whether we deserve them. If they can come to believe in a nonpunishing, nonjudgmental God, it can help them accept a diagnosis and a plan of treatment. There is a kind of peace that comes from finding a God that helps them to accept what is happening to them, rather than hoping for a magical, rescuing God.*
>
> *My own understanding of spirituality is that it is not a search for an outside source of strength but rather a call to go deeply within ourselves, tapping our unconscious resources. I teach my patients self-hypnosis—which creates the same effect as meditation—a state that allows us to have a relationship with that inner resource. In this hypnotic state, healing is promoted, whatever the outcome of the illness."*
> —Valerie Johns, *M.A., M.F.T.*

The result of my illness has not been that I've become more religious, but I have become more self-aware. I still probably go to therapy more often than I go to church, but more than anything my desire has been to discover the lessons I was meant to learn from this crisis. They say danger and opportunity are present in every crisis, and I found that to be true for me. The danger has passed, but the opportunities continue to present themselves every day. Faith and spirituality played a different role in the lives of each of the moms I met *before* they were sick and the same is true for how their illness impacted their spirituality and their view of the role faith or religion played in their lives.

◆ *Mothers' Wisdom* ◆

I've been practicing zazen (Zen Buddhist sitting meditation) and studying Buddhism for several years after twenty-five years of not identifying with any religion whatsoever. On my second day in the hospital, as they were doing a lot of diagnostic procedures to see how much damage had been done to my lungs (thankfully, very little) and heart (none) by the embolism, I thought I was handling all this very well, but in the middle of a cardiac ultrasound, as I was watching my own heart on the monitor, I was seized by panic as the level of the danger I was in suddenly became clear. After ten minutes of sheer terror, though, I was able to clear my mind a little and let go of the fear. That left just the stark fact of my illness, the fact that I was in grave danger and might die—or not—at any moment. But I saw it with great clarity and calm, and had a strong sense of acceptance—except for the fear and sadness I felt for my husband and children— whatever happened was going to happen, and that was that. I am extremely glad, of course, that I didn't die, but now when I hear or read the evening chant that comes at the end of some Buddhist services, reminding us that life and death are of supreme importance, that death could come at any time, and that we must not waste our lives, it comes with a much greater sense of urgency and clarity than ever before when these ideas seemed purely theoretical. I hadn't thought of it before, but I had my husband bring in my little pocket Buddha (brass, about one to one and a half inches high) and I kept it on my hospital tray. I also tried to keep up with my daily sitting—there's certainly plenty of free time for that in a hospital!—and found that it helped me (and continues to help me) not to be overwhelmed by what was happening or what might happen.—Nancy

My spiritual life has definitely changed. I have always been a big prayer person, but I rely upon praying more. It seems like I am asking for my guidance with my health in the way eating better, taking care of myself better, and to get better educated with my disease. I have seen some of my prayers answered as well. I have taken classes to help me understand my disease with regard to diet and exercise. I still pray for daily help!—Shelley

It's interesting to think about faith and my disease. I often think that I am blessed in a way to have been forced to slow down. To stop and look at what I do have. I have to be more mindful of things, of the next step, of where I put something or what I was doing. I am so appreciative of all that I have. I would say that I have a strong faith and look forward to an hour a week at church to contemplate or meditate on life and what needs attention. And be reminded that I can start fresh and make another go at making things as right as possible. —Grace

As for spirituality, I think motherhood has made me more spiritual. I found I had to really develop my faith when I learned I was pregnant—hoping I could manage my health to provide my babies with the best possible starts, trusting in physicians, etc. wouldn't have been enough. After nearly losing my older son when I went into eclamptic seizures, I am constantly reminding myself that the worst day with them is better than the best day without them—that I have been blessed.—Catherine

I felt very strong emotions when I was at church during my illness. I almost found it unbearable to be there. I would cry and cry and cry when I was in church. It was a place where I felt I could really be who I needed to be. That was wonderful on the one hand; on the other hand, I sometimes just stayed away. I have often heard it said that you can tell when something is really wrong in someone's life because they stop coming to church. I used to think that meant that they were doubting. In my case, it was that I felt so fragile—so human—at church, because the presence of God felt so strong. I didn't pray any more when I was sick than I did otherwise. I felt like all my actions were, in some ways, a kind of prayer. I felt so close to God that I didn't feel like I even needed to pray. It was very odd. Friends of all kinds asked if they could put me on the prayer lists at their church—Baptists and Catholics and Episcopalians and Mormons. I always said *of course.* One of my best friends wanted me to have a hands-on blessing from her Mormon bishops. It's a very intimate prayer, where a group of elder men in their church gather around and lay hands on your head, and pray for specific things that come to them. I agreed, and I loved it. It was very moving to be part of a prayer ritual that wasn't mine. It made me feel the universality of God and prayer, and the many ways that we all try to connect.—Jennie

I've never been spiritual and that hasn't changed since I got sick. I've never said "Why me?" or felt angry that someone or something did this to me and I deserve an explanation. My mom has broken down on several occasions and said 'I wish you had something to fall back on, some faith,' and I suppose there have been a few times when I've been really low, in a lot of pain or fear and I've thought that would be convenient, but that has been about the extent of it. When I had cancer, I really fought that disease, but when I got fibromyalgia, I had to learn to stop fighting, because that only makes it worse. It took me at least a year to learn that and get to a place of acceptance. I guess some people might call that a kind of faith, but I just consider it learning about what works and what doesn't, and directing my energy in the most productive way I can.—Stephanie

Once I got over my disappointment that I didn't have a Hollywood-style encounter with God and my fear that this somehow meant that God was displeased with me, I began to see Him everywhere. He showed up when I had to hire a new nanny, and he sent a real-life angel to apply for the job. He appeared when Justus had the courage to identify the "virus on my spirit" and thus spark my interest in discovering the meaning of what had happened and how it might change our lives. He was there again when cutbacks at work threatened my job and gave me the courage to quit and begin work on this book. He continues to show up in the words and warm embrace of my children as we heal the wounds and calm the fears that my illness stirred up.

But more than anything, my higher power has revealed itself through the women who appear in the pages of this book. Sick moms are often scared, angry, and exhausted but they are also in what can only be described as a state of grace.

They have an inner peace and a broad view. In many cases, they've seen the worst and survived. In others, they know more struggles lie ahead but they're fortified for the battle so they spend little time worrying about when it will come or what it will bring. Sick moms are wise, caring, and balanced. They don't take things for granted and they know God—whether that's through walks on the beach, Sabbath trips to the synagogue, or in the embrace of a friend.

So, while I didn't see God when my heart stopped, She was there.

My heart started again and I have seen Her every day since.

From Cacophony
to Symphony

I asked my doctors about what happened during the thirty-five seconds my heart had stopped and they explained that I wasn't "gone long enough" for the God/bright light/floating thing to have happened. Part of my body, my heart, had shut down, but the rest of me was still "alive" and the cacophony was my system's urgent attempt to figure out what was wrong and fix it.

I asked a psychic about it and she said that it was the sound of a door opening and closing. This could mean one of two things, she said. One interpretation was that it was the door between life and death and I was standing in the threshold deciding whether to pass through. The other, she said, was that the door opened to let more spirit, peace, and possibilities into my life and then it closed so I could wake up and move on with new awareness and new promise. I liked the sound of that.

PART IV

• • • • • • • •

HOW YOUR ILLNESS
AFFECTS YOUR FUTURE

A DOZEN THINGS
I LEARNED FROM
BEING A SICK MOM

⊚　⊚　⊚　⊚　⊚　⊚　⊚　⊚　⊚　⊚　⊚　⊚　⊚　⊚　⊚　⊚

Rather than thinking of illness as disaster, we can think of it as a powerful and useful message . . . that there is something to be looked at within our consciousness, something to be recognized, acknowledged, and healed. It may indicate that there is something about the way we are living that needs to be changed.

—SHAKTI GAWAIN,
　Reflections in the Light

When I finally stopped running from my story and began to delve into the "How comes?" and "What nows?" of the experience, I expected some big answers. The experience of being a sick mom is so challenging and traumatic that it seemed to me it needed to add up to something. And the good news is, it did—and it does.

Whether a mom is sick for a few months, few years, or even for the rest of her life, it seems only fair that she should get something in return. Wouldn't it be great, having gone through this crisis, if she (if *we*) could say when it was over that it was worth it because of the lessons learned? At the very least, I'd hope we would be able to point out a few good things that came from it.

I have gotten to this point. It has taken most of the four years since my illness for this to be true, but I can now say that I am grateful for what happened and that my life is better today because of it. Indeed, I don't know if I could have or would have learned the lessons taught to me by this experience any other way—and I needed to learn them.

Here they are in a nutshell, and then again below in more detail. May they resonate for you or point you in the right direction.

1. Be sick so you can get better.
2. Ask for help.
3. Don't be picky
4. Break your rules.
5. Be honest with your kids.
6. Involve your partner.
7. Find someone to talk to.
8. Go slow.
9. Say no.
10. Put yourself first.
11. See old things in a new way.
12. Never take your health for granted.

Lessons are very personal so these might not all speak to you, but they say that the universe provides us with the teachers we need when we need them. My illness was my teacher and yours may be too.

Here's a bit more about the lessons that were most significant to me.

1) Be sick so you can get better.

The sooner you give in and let yourself be sick, the faster you'll heal emotionally and physically. This means naps, healthy food, taking your medicine, sitting on the couch while everyone waits on you hand and foot. If you have to, pretend your child is the one who has your disease and think about how you'd care for her. With this in mind, care for yourself in the same way. And you can cry, mope, and stomp your feet. Being sick is no fun and you don't have to pretend it's okay.

2) Ask for help.

This is simultaneously the most important yet hardest lesson to learn for women in general, and sick moms in particular. You've been a doer and a giver. Become an asker and receiver. Ask for help with anything that can be done by someone else and save your energy for the one thing that you alone can do—get better!

3) Don't be picky.

It doesn't matter how the laundry is folded or whether the friend who's offered to take your kids to school is always late. It doesn't matter if your husband burns the grilled cheese or your daughter wears snow boots to school every day. The point is that you've asked for help and it's arrived. Now you have to be grateful; be quiet and accept what's being offered.

4) Break your rules.

As we parent, we develop a set of unwritten but inviolable rules that govern everything from what we serve our kids to eat to how long they're allowed to use their PlayStation. Some of the rules are hand-me-downs, inherited from our parents. Others are fresh and possibly a reaction to how we were raised and our ideas about doing it better with our kids. Regardless, we've got systems and protocols in place—but when we're sick it's time to forget them. The *only* thing that matters is that we're focused on our healing. Everything else will take care of itself. Introduce your family to "crazy days," serve cereal for dinner, and let the dust bunnies roam.

5) Be honest with your kids.

Your kids deserve to know what's going on and they need to hear it from you. If you've got cancer or another potentially fatal disease, be prepared to answer their questions about death. If you've got a chronic condition such as multiple sclerosis or diabetes, they deserve to know that mommy doesn't always know how she's going to feel day to day and that some days are really hard. If you're going through testing, let them know that the doctors are trying to help mommy find out what's wrong. Thinking that we're sparing them by not talking to them does not work. Kids have an acute sixth sense and know when something is amiss. They'll be more frightened if they have to try to figure it out by themselves.

6) Involve your partner.

Illness puts great strain on your primary relationship. Your roles and the normal division of labor will be turned upside down and that may breed guilt and resentment. It may be tempting to talk of nothing else but the details of your treatments and medical condition, or spend your few spare moments talking about how all this is affecting the kids. But talking to each other about your feelings and fears is critical.

7) Find someone to talk to.

No matter how much is going on with your physical health, you can be sure that your mental health is in just as much turmoil. The journey from in-charge I-can-do-it mom to cancel-everything I-need-to-rest mom is an emotional one. You've got doctors helping you heal your body; you need professionals to help you with your spirit too. Go see a counselor or attend a group session led by one. Even if you only go a few times, giving yourself this gift will yield inspiration and insight that will help greatly.

8) Go slow.

Remember the stories about the pumpkin patch, the lone casserole, and my "all-important" lunch meeting with my boss *four days after surgery?* Well, these are but three examples of what *not* to do and how you can derail your healing. So, my advice is to *go slow* when you're deciding about when to return to your usual activities, because people aren't expecting to see you, but once they *do*, they'll assume you're available and ready to take on projects and assignments that may be too taxing.

9) Say no.

When you do reemerge, your only protection is going to be this one little word. Just because you "always" volunteered at the kids school in the past or your boss could "always" count on you to work late doesn't mean that this can continue. Women (and especially moms) are notoriously bad at saying 'no,' but for sick and recovering moms, it is a must—and you don't even have to explain why. Like asking for help, you can start with the small things (like "No, I'm sorry I can't watch Emma today after school.") and move to bigger things ("I'm flattered that you're considering me for that promotion but I'd like to take my name off the list because I want to spend more time with my family."). Being sick gives you the license to say 'no' that you didn't think you had. Don't squander it.

10) Put yourself first.

No matter what decision you have to make, you and your needs must be taken into consideration. Even if it's something as simple as feeding the kids leftovers rather than stopping at the market on your way home from work when you're dead tired and you know the place is going to be packed, you need to think about what's good for you. Before we got sick, we may have rarely considered our needs as we went about the business of planning and executing activities at work and home. No more. Now when we give, we give from our overflow. Sometimes things will go our way, sometimes things won't, but at least we'll know the difference and at least we'll have experienced the balance we're striving for.

11) See old things in a new way.

Many mothers approach life as if they are beholden to everyone but themselves. We think we're limited in what we can and cannot do because so many people are counting on us for so much. We feel overwhelmed with obligations and bereft of options. We feel trapped. In truth and fact the only true obligations we have is to care for ourselves and our families—and we have plenty of options as to how we'll do so.

12) Never take your health for granted.

When you're a sick mom you learn once and for all that there is no "mom immunity" and that we're just as likely to get sick as anybody else. We also learn that our health can no longer take a backseat to our kids' health, husband's health, and the dog's trip to the vet. Moms have to make (and keep) their annual appointments with the OB-GYN and internist. Moms need to monitor their cholesterol, blood pressure, and blood sugar levels. Moms need to check for lumps monthly and have a Pap smear annually. Moms need to get their sleep, eat right, and exercise. No excuses, no whining about how busy we are. As sick moms we have lived diagnosis and treatment; now we can preach and practice prevention.

WHAT SICK MOMS CAN TEACH THE WORLD

. . . or at Least the Other Moms They Know

◦ ◦ ◦ ◦ ◦ ◦ ◦ ◦ ◦ ◦ ◦ ◦ ◦ ◦ ◦

Healing is a matter of time, but it is also sometimes a matter of opportunity.

—HIPPOCRATES

Whether you suffer from a onetime acute illness or live with a chronic, debilitating condition, the experience of being a sick mom is one that changes you forever.

If, like Andrea or Sue, you had a serious accident that left you temporarily bedridden and unable to carry your kids, drive a car, or even climb a flight of stairs, you'll never take your independence for granted again. If like Paula, Nancy, or Jackie, you had a debilitating onetime crisis, you recall with awe and amazement the friends who appeared out of thin air to pitch in to see you through and you're now keenly attuned to the needs of other people (especially other moms) and find ways to give back through giving to them.

If, like Shelley, Catherine, Stephanie, Melissa, Grace, and Darcy, your illness is ongoing and your goal is to manage it within the joys and pressures of your day-to-day life, you crave "good days" when mommy has enough energy and mobility to build sand castles and stay up late watching movies and munching popcorn. You also prepare for "bad days" when you have to stay in bed and hope that your kids will be patient and remember the good days.

If like Jennie, Jennifer, Marty, Jacqueline, Fern, Mary Ellen, and Cathy, you battled cancer and call yourself a survivor but never say you're cured, you go about your "normal" routine knowing that in an instant life can be turned upside down and it's imperative to look for and find joy in the little things.

If, like me, you were sick and denied it and were scared but didn't tell a soul, you continue to mine the experience for all it's worth and marvel as much in your emotional healing as your physical recovery.

If getting sick in the midst of grocery lists and homework assignments, dirty diapers and college applications, climbing the career ladder and maintaining a loving marriage teaches us anything, it teaches us that bad things happen to good people, life is not always fair, and we're capable of much more than we ever dreamed. Getting sick provides perspective, motivation, and wisdom.

We learn, as one mom said, "There is no 'why.' It just is," and we look for ways to move forward without forgetting where we've been and what it meant.

The New
To-Do List

During the course of writing this book, I got sick several times. Nothing serious, just your run-of-the-mill series of headcolds, headaches, allergy attacks, and the occasional flu that come with the territory when you've got school-age kids. What was different, however, is how I reacted to these all-too-familiar maladies. For the first time, I took care of myself.

Mind you, it didn't happen all at once, and more than once my mom, husband, or girlfriends had to remind me to take it easy. "Isn't that what your book is all about?" they would inquire. "Aren't you telling women they need to put themselves first and learn how to ask for help?"

"Yes," I would reply, and then review my day's to-do list, looking for anything that could be considered optional, rather than obligatory. When I looked at it with the same critical eye I advise in this book, I invariably found that there was very little that I absolutely had to do and a lot of things that I simply planned on doing.

Using a kind of "sick moms' litmus test," I was able to immediately whittle away at the list and carve out some time for a nap, a doctor's appointment, or a steamy bath to ease my symptoms. And sometimes, oftentimes, that meant calling someone and telling them that I would be unable to keep my commitment or previously scheduled engagement. And over time I learned something here too.

Most of the time when you change plans or have to renege on a promise, you don't have to make excuses or even have much of an explanation.

I would be all prepared to recite my tale of woe about my 101-degree temperature or my aching head to the person on the other end of the line, and found that after I uttered the words, "I'm sorry, I'm not feeling well and am not going to be able to make it," or something to that effect, they usually didn't need any more information. I could almost hear them moving on mentally as they wished me well and began to plot their next move now that they knew I wouldn't be bringing the cupcakes, presenting at the meeting, or _____ (fill in the blank.)

This has been one of the most important lessons of my illness and recovery and is the one that stands the best chance of helping every mom, be she well, sick, or on the road to recovery.

When we're really sick, with cancer, heart disease, or a flare-up of MS symptoms, everything really does shut down and, for the most part, everyone gets along. Armed with this knowledge, this little "sick mom's secret," we can approach all our days differently and see that our long list of things to do is nothing more than a rough plan that can be altered or jettisoned at any moment. The reason can be a sore throat, sprained ankle, or abnormal Pap smear—and when we get really good, the reason can be a massage appointment that takes precedence over the PTA meeting or a spur-of-the-moment lunch date with our husband that commands the time we'd earlier allotted to scouting locations for the office holiday party.

✔ TRY THIS

CHOICE—Write this word at the top of your daily to-do list and remember the days and weeks when not only were the things on the list not done but the lists were not even made. When you are really sick and have no choice, you put yourself first. Try doing that when you're just a little under the weather—or better yet when you feel on top of the world.

What Sick Moms Can Teach the World

Many people—especially women, and even more so, mothers—move through life reacting to circumstances and doing things as if they had no say in the matter. We take promotions, agree to sing in the choir at church, and tell the kids they can get a puppy, often without even considering if it's really what we want. We're so concerned about hurting people's feelings and letting people down that we lose track of what's best for us.

Sick moms cannot afford to do that.

Even if we're quite expert at the juggling act that is mother-hood, it's impossible to follow through on every responsibility when we're sick and getting better. We have to let things fall apart just enough so that we can put ourselves back together. And when we let that happen, even for the little things, we discover something truly amazing. Everything is just fine.

Meetings go on without us, kids discover the joy of owning a hamster (instead of a dog), the fund-raiser goes off without a hitch, and other people get the kudos. We learn that we're not indispensable, and while this may bruise our ego, it's a great boon to our health.

Getting sick is a break in the action from which we can emerge with a keener sense of who we are and what's important. No matter how we did it before, what we were like, and what people have come to expect from us, we can do it completely differently once we've been sick.

Illness hands us a new set of rules to live by—and we can share these lessons with others so maybe they can learn them without ever having to be sick.

This is the gift sick moms can give to the world. That is, if they first give it to themselves.

PART V

. . . .

RESOURCES

WHERE TO TURN FOR MORE HELP

When you're a sick mom, you're typically short on time and long on questions. There are hundreds (likely, thousands) of books, Web sites, and associations that can educate you about your condition, guide you through the emotional ups and downs, and lend a hand in helping you understand how your children might be reacting to your illness and what you can do to help. *Cereal for Dinner* does not seek to replace any of these, but seeks to be an additional voice, a mom's voice, in the ongoing discussion you're likely engaged in related to being *in*firmed and *in* charge at the same time.

A complete list of all the resources available to you would be longer than this entire book. Even a comprehensive list is tricky to put together because you're bound to forget something that someone needs. Understanding the limits of what fits (both literally and figuratively) in a resource section, I have provided the following list of publications I've read, Web sites I've visited, and organizations that I can recommend or that have been recommended to me. It just scratches the surface, but my goal here is to keep it simple and keep you smiling.

Good Places to Start

Centers for Disease Control and Prevention, 1600 Clifton Rd., Atlanta, GA 30333. 800-311-3435. *www.cdc.gov*

Johns Hopkins Hospital and Health System, 600 Wolfe St., Baltimore, MD 21287. 410-955-5000. *www.hopkinsmedicine.org*

Mayo Clinic, Locations in Arizona, Florida, Minnesota. *www.mayoclinic.org*

WebMD, *www.webmd.com.*

The "Big Kahuna" Associations

American Cancer Society, 1599 Clifton Rd. NE, Atlanta, GA 30329. 800-ACS-2345. *www.cancer.org*

American Diabetes Association, 1701 N. Beauregard St., Alexandria, VA 22311. 800-342-2383. *www.diabetes.org*

American Heart Association, 7272 Greenville Ave., Dallas, TX 75231. 800-242-8721. *www.americanheart.org*

American Lung Association, 61 Broadway, 6th Floor, New York, NY 10006. 212-315-8700. *www.lungusa.org*

National Multiple Sclerosis Society, 733 Third Ave., New York, NY 10017. 800-FIGHTMS (800-344-4867). *www.nmss.org*

Susan G. Komen Breast Cancer Foundation, 5005 LBJ Freeway, Suite 250, Dallas, TX 75244. *www.komen.org*

Lesser Known But Equally Important Organizations

Diabetic Mommy, *www.diabeticmommy.com*

MSMoms, (support group for moms with multiple sclerosis) 9331 Rocky Lane, Orangevale, CA 95622. *www.msmoms.com*

National Women's Health Information Center (sponsored by the U.S. Dept. of Health and Human Services), 8550 Arlington Blvd., Suite 300, Fairfax, VA 22031. 800-994-WOMAN (800-944-9662). *www.4woman.gov*

Women's Cancer Network, 401 N. Michigan Ave., Chicago, IL 60611. 312-644-6610. *www.wcn.org*

Parents with Disabilities, *www.disabledparents.net*

Yes, Virginia, There Is a Group for You Too

American Chronic Pain Association, PO Box 850, Rocklin, CA 95677. 800-533-3231. *www.theacpa.org*

Chronic Fatigue and Immune Dysfunction Syndrome Association of America, PO Box 220398, Charlotte, NC 28222. 704-365-2343. *www.cfids.org*

Fibromyalgia Network, PO Box 31750, Tucson, AZ 85751. 800-853-2929. *www.fmnetnews.com*

HysterSisters, Inc. (support for women considering or recovering from a hysterectomy), 2436 S. I-35 East, Denton, TX 76205. 940-898-0070. *www.hystersisters.com*

Interstitial Cystitis Association. 110 N. Washington St., Suite 340, Rockville, MD 20850. 800-HELP-ICA. *www.ichelp.com*

Irritable Bowel Syndrome Association, 1440 Whalley Ave., New Haven, CT 06515. *www.ibsassociation.org*

Lupus Foundation of America, 2000 L Street NW, Washington, D.C. 20036. 202-349-1155. *www.lupus.org*

National Migraine Association, 113 S. Saint Asaph, Suite 300, Alexandria, VA 22314. 703-739-9384. *www.migraines.org*

www.Yahoo.com and www.Google.com—type in key words and begin a search for whatever ails you.

Where to Turn When You're at Your Wits' End

About Psychotherapy, *www.aboutpsychotherapy.com*

American Psychological Association, 750 First St. NE, Washington, D.C. 20002. 800-964-2000 for referral. *www.apa.org*

Find a Therapist, Inc., 515 N. 16th St., Suite A-116, Phoenix, AZ 85016. 800-865-0685. *www.find-a-therapist.com*

Local hospitals and chapters of the "big kahuna" associations offer peer and support groups filled with people who understand.

Helping You Help Your Kids (and Your Spouse)

Web sites:

KidsKonnected. Support group for kids who have a parent with cancer. *www.kidskonnected.com.*

Kids in Crisis. On-line help for teens. *www.geocities.com/heartland/bluffs/5400/depression*

Rainbows. On-line support and resources for children grieving or dealing with a life-altering crisis. *www.rainbows.org*

Well Spouse Foundation. Resources and assistance for caretakers. *www.wellspouse.org*

Books:

Can I Still Kiss You: Answering Your Kids Questions about Cancer, by Neil Russell (Health Communications, Inc., 2001)

How to Help Your Children Through a Parent's Serious Illness, by Kathleen McCue. (St. Martin's Press, 1996)

It Won't Hurt Forever: Guiding Your Child Through Trauma. by Dr. Peter Levine, audio recording produced by Sounds True, *www.soundstrue.com*, 2001.

When a Parent Has Cancer, by Dr. Wendy S. Harpham (Harper Collins, 1997)

When You Want to Try Something Totally Different

Alternative Therapies in Health and Medicine, 169 Saxony Rd., Suite 104, Encinitas, CA 92024. 866-828-2962. *www.alternative-therapies.com*

Holistic.com. Find a massage therapist, acupuncturist, or chiropractor in your city; enjoy a four-minute streaming video yoga class; and more. *www.holistic.com.*

Some Books That Help

The Cherished Self, by Michelle Morris-Spieker

Kitchen Table Wisdom, by Naomi Remen, M.D

The Victoria's Secret Catalog Never Stops Coming and Other Lessons I Learned from Breast Cancer, by Jennie Nash

When Life Becomes Precious, by Elise NeeDell Babcock

When Bad Things Happen to Good People, by Harold Kushner

Women's Bodies, Women's Wisdom, by Christiane Northrup, M.D.

ABOUT THE AUTHOR

When Kristine Breese was eight-years-old, she walked door-to-door in her first political campaign. Granola bars and raisins fueled her march. When she went to Capitol Hill as a congressional intern, she subsisted on chicken wings and shrimp cocktail. At UCLA, microwave popcorn and Dominoes Pizza were de rigueur, and in journalism school her roommate's Toll House cookies were a staple. Never, however, has a menu so suited her situation as when she became a sick mom and started serving cereal for dinner. Today Breese works as a writer, consultant, and motivational speaker, and has found that you don't need to be sick to pour dinner from a box. She lives in Los Angeles with her husband, two children, and a black Labrador named Hollywood.

www.kristinebreese.com